Product Ma for Hospitals

Organizing for Profitability

James C. Folger and E. Preston Gee

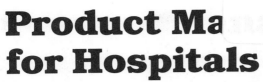

American Hospital Publishing, Inc.,
a wholly owned subsidiary
of the American Hospital Association

The views in this book are those of the authors.

Library of Congress Cataloging-in-Publication Data

Folger, James C.
  Product management for hospitals.

  Includes bibliographies.
  1. Hospitals—Marketing—Management. 2. Product
management. I. Gee, Erin Preston. II. Title. [DNLM:
1. Financial Management. 2. Hospital Administration—
economics. 3. Marketing of Health Services.
WX 157 F664p]
RA965.5.F64 1987 362.1'1'0688   87-12616
ISBN 1-55648-007-5

Catalog no. 136102

Text set in Bookman Light
3.0M—7/87-0182
2.0M—2/89-0233
Audrey Kaufman, Project Editor
Wayne S. Brown, Managing Editor
Peggy DuMais, Production Coordinator
Marcia Vecchione, Designer
Brian W. Schenk, Books Division Director

Contents

List of Tables and Figures

Tables

Figures

Preface

The hospital industry is currently operating in an extremely competitive environment, where some will win and many others will lose. In 1981, Jeff Goldsmith examined the framework in which hospitals would have to compete as the industry is transformed from a regulatory to a competitive environment. He concluded that many would not survive in this strange, new environment (*Can Hospitals Survive? The New Competitive Health Care Market*. Homewood, IL: Dow Jones-Irwin, 1981).

Our response to Goldsmith is that hospitals **can survive** through product-line management—an idea whose time, if not already here, is rapidly approaching. The innovators in health care thinking, planning, and organization are beginning to come out in strong support for the concepts of product management. In late 1986, Leland Kaiser, the well-regarded health care educator and futurist, wrote: "Product management is the type of management needed in a high-tech marketplace. Physicians, nurses, and allied health professionals will spend increasing amounts of time serving on production teams designing and developing new products" (*Healthcare Forum* Nov./Dec. 1986).

Without competition, there would be little need to consider alternatives to existing management structures. Product management made sense for other industries for the same reasons it currently makes sense for health care; namely, by managing products as separate business entities, one can compete more effectively in the marketplace. The hospital has become too complex to compete as a single entity; administration simply cannot find the time nor devote the energy to each of the service components. Product management solves this problem because each of the individual services/programs competes separately; that is, the parts become greater than the whole.

Product Management for Hospitals was written for hospital marketers, CEOs, and CFOs who are looking for ways to compete more effectively in the marketplace. It will also serve as a text for students learning about new methods of management in health care settings. The book provides the reader with a basic understanding of product-line management and how it can be applied in the health care environment; it sets up a framework for the development, implementation, and review of the product-management strategy in hospitals. Individual chapters illustrate how product management has evolved in the health care industry, what product-line management means, how to find a product manager, how to set up a management team, how to measure results, how to review strategies, and, most important, how to make it happen.

No health care organization can remain passive in these exciting but turbulent times and expect to survive intact. Product-line management offers the means whereby a hospital can meet the challenges of today and emerge as a winner tomorrow.

Acknowledgments

We would like to acknowledge the many people who have made valuable contributions to the book. First, a special thanks to our marketing counterparts throughout the country who have shared experiences and insights and who have helped validate the viability of product management. We are similarly appreciative of the administration and middle management at Sacred Heart General Hospital for their interest and support in adopting the product-line concept.

Our sincere thanks also to Louise Shimmel who deciphered our scribbling in typing the manuscript, proving that the translation of ancient hieroglyphics is relatively easy compared to these authors' contemporary cursives.

Finally, a debt of gratitude to our wives Susan Folger and Janice Gee for their continued support and positive reinforcement throughout the development of this book.

About the Authors

James C. Folger is currently president of Northwest Healthcare Consulting, Eugene, Oregon, a consulting practice that focuses on business/marketing planning, program development, and product-line management in hospitals. Prior to establishing Northwest Healthcare, Folger was director of planning and marketing at Sacred Heart General Hospital, Eugene; marketing development manager at Humana, Inc., Louisville, KY; and had nine years of marketing experience with consumer and industrial product goods at Monsanto Company and H.J. Heinz Company. He received a master's degree in business administration from the University of Michigan, Ann Arbor.

E. Preston Gee is director of marketing and strategic planning, Sacred Heart General Hospital, Eugene, Oregon, where he coordinated the first product management teams and developed business plans for cancer, cardiology, and home health product lines. Prior to joining Sacred Heart General Hospital, Gee was marketing manager of educational software and senior marketing research analyst at Fisher-Price Toys Division, Quaker Oats Company, East Aurora, New York. He received a master's degree in business administration from Brigham Young University, Provo, Utah.

Chapter 1

Introduction

---

*"All things must change
To Something new, something strange."*

—Longfellow

The Process of Evolution

In a presentation he made before the Society for Hospital Planning of the American Hospital Association in 1984, Philip Kotler compared the evolution of planning and marketing in American industry with that in hospitals.[1] As shown in table 1, hospitals have been 20 years behind the business community in using sales and marketing but are gradually closing the gap with strategic planning and management.

Kotler defines each of the phases as follows:

- **Sales planning** consists of formulating a plan for selling an existing product or service, including its possible target markets, prices, distribution, and promotion support.
- **Marketing planning** consists of analyzing the market opportunities facing a particular business unit, researching the target markets and their needs, developing attractive marketing offers, formulating winning strategies, and designing, implementing, and controlling cost-effective marketing tactics.
- **Strategic planning** is the managerial process of developing and maintaining a viable fit between the organization's objectives and resources and its environmental opportunities. The job of strategic planning is to design the organization in such a way that it consists of a healthy balance

Table 1. Evolution of Marketing and Planning in Industry vs. Hospitals

Marketing/Planning Approach	Era First Introduced	
	Industry	Hospitals
Sales planning	1950	1970
Marketing planning	1960	1980
Strategic planning	1970	1985
Strategic management	1980	1990

of businesses that achieve the return-risk goals of the organization.

- **Strategic management** consists of line managers taking responsibility for assessing the future of their businesses, developing long-term goals as to where to take their businesses, and formulating effective strategies for reaching their goals. Operations management, on the other hand, consists of line managers setting goals for the year and carefully controlling their activities and costs to achieve these goals.

What we can look forward to in 1990 is a strategic management process that pushes decision making down to lower levels. What Kotler has described as "strategic management" comes very close to a definition of the role of the product manager, and we would propose that organizational evolution may occur as follows:

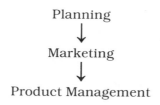

Planning
↓
Marketing
↓
Product Management

Product management represents the next step after a marketing adaptation, because it offers a more sophisticated means to operate and manage a business in an increasingly competitive environment. **The essence of product management exists in breaking down and operating services as profit centers unto themselves,** which we will explore in greater depth in chapters 2 and 3. This breakup is already occurring, and the losers will be those who try to stand in the way of the inevitable in the hope that things will return to the way they used to be.

The Future Is Yet to Come

When Arthur Andersen & Co. completed its study of *Health Care in the 1990s* in conjunction with the American College of Hospital Administrators in 1984,[2] all signs pointed to the advent of product management:

> To compete effectively, each hospital must analyze its market, customers and competitors, as well as its competitive strengths and weaknesses, in order to develop and deliver competitive services and products.

Further:

> Providers must segment their markets, *introduce product line management into their delivery system,* and develop those services which they can deliver most cost-effectively and profitably.

One of the major changes wrought by the diagnosis-related groups (DRGs) and the advent of competition is the realization that the hospital can no longer be managed as a total entity, because the task has become too complex. In the face of shrinking inpatient volumes and a tightening of the reimbursement belt, mistakes are no longer tolerated that previously could have been absorbed by the entity or passed on to employers and the government in higher costs or charges. Product management offers the means whereby the hospital, in effect, becomes many small hospitals, each with its own distinct identity, management, and goals.

Small, Flexible, and a Winner

The onset of cost controls and diminishing funds for capital investment has focused more scrutiny on the purchase of new technology. The needs of the market must now be addressed and the question asked, "If I were spending my own money, would I compete successfully with their technology?"

The change in approach is worthy of an example. Most large hospitals (as of this writing) have purchased or are planning to purchase a magnetic resonance imager (MRI). The most popular version is the one with a superconducting 1.5 tesla magnet. The magnet is so powerful that it needs shielding to a radius of 40 feet and costs upwards of $2 million.

We talked to an entrepreneur who had started a diagnostic imaging center and asked his opinion of the hospitals' rush to add this new technology. He commented that he felt smug every time he heard about a hospital adding one of these big, new 1.5 tesla MRIs, because he has a low-cost .15 tesla MRI that needs very little shielding and can do 95 percent of what the big machines do. His small, flexible approach is the ticket to success in today's changing environment. True, in five years there may be new diagnostic procedures that demand a superstrength magnet, but by then the cost of the equipment may be half of what it is today. Because hospitals no longer have unlimited access to capital, it is important to allocate resources in the most effective manner.

Down with Bureaucracy

These are exciting times for those who adapt well to change. However, many administrators may suffer from the "future shock" that Alvin Toffler discussed in his now-classic book about what happens to people when they are overwhelmed by change.[3] The variety of choices and accelerated time frames for decision making can very easily lead to overload. But, as Toffler suggests, the problem is not how to suppress change but how to manage it. To quote him:

> This typically bureaucratic arrangement is ideally suited to solving routine problems at a moderate pace. But when things speed up, or the problems cease to be routine, chaos often breaks loose.

Toffler comments that an "ad-hocracy" of temporary systems will be formed to take the place of bureaucracy and references Warren Bennis, a social psychologist and professor of industrial management, who predicted that in 25 to 50 years we will all participate in the end of bureaucracy. Toffler states that "executives and managers in this system will function as coordinators between the various transient work teams. They will be skilled in understanding the jargon of different groups of specialists, and they will communicate across groups, translating and interpreting the language of one into the language of another. People in this system will, according to Bennis, 'be differentiated not vertically, according to rank and role, but flexibly and functionally, according to skill and professional training.'"

What Toffler and Bennis describe is the prototype for a product manager of a matrix team in the new hospital environment.

Changing Times

No doubt these are difficult times for health care professionals. The veterans have seen more change in the last 3 years than in the preceding 30.

The Administrator's Perspective

A recent survey by Touche Ross revealed that 43 percent of the administrators surveyed felt that their hospitals were at risk of failure within the next five years.[4] It is not surprising that the majority of the 43 percent presided over hospitals with fewer than 200 beds in rural communities.

No wonder, then, that administrators are grasping at straws and that, in the process, some are making unwise managerial decisions. "When in unfamiliar waters," wrote the sage, "grab any lifeline, whether familiar or not."

The Physician's Perspective

Then there are the physicians. What may already have been a testy situation has been exacerbated by the recent changes in the health care setting. In many respects, the only profession experiencing more volatility than that of the CEO is that of the doctor.

Doctors suddenly find their previously predictable world spoiled with three-letter words such as HMO, PPO, PPS, and the like. More medical graduates are accepting salaried positions. In 1985, 12-1/2 percent of U.S. physicians were on salary. Significantly, of those doctors on salary, 40 percent were 37 years of age or younger. Pouring salt on the wound, more and more hospitals are "practicing medicine" by offering "urgicenters," "surgicenters," walk-in clinics, and imaging facilities that seem to be in direct competition with doctors.

Consumer Sovereignty

Finally, there is the new breed of consumer—the patients. Not only do contemporary consumers complain that costs are exorbitant, but they have heard the "have it your way" message so long that they actually believe it applies to hospitals. Hospitals used to be places where one accepted the care given, not demanded the care expected. These days, if a couple doesn't have a padded rocker in the room, oriental rugs on the floor, piped-in music (Dolby stereo), and a champagne dinner afterward, the birth of a child is a second-class experience.

Whereas some hospital employees have embraced these changes with excitement and enthusiasm, many find the upheaval extremely frustrating. As one nurse put it, "If I had wanted to be a flight attendant, I wouldn't have gone to nursing school."

A Search for Precedents in the Service Industries

Certainly, the hospital industry is not alone in the change game. Airlines, banks, and hotels have all undergone similar changes as they entered the world of competition. The airlines, for instance, have undergone rapid shifts. Twenty years ago the skies were not friendly, and the "only way to fly" was any airplane one could find, not a particular airline.

Not too long ago, the only recognizable difference among banks was the gift one received for making a deposit. Now there are automatic tellers, money market accounts, NOW accounts, and a host of accepted additions. Even in this highly regulated industry, there is considerable effort to distinguish one institution from its competition.

The hotel industry is often cited as a predominant predecessor of hospitals. Remember when a hotel was a hotel was a hotel and the only ones with pools were in Florida, California, and Arizona? There were no discernible differences among Hyatts, Hiltons, Marriotts, and Holiday Inns.

The way these industries have adopted, and adapted to, the changes provides an insight for hospitals. As mentioned, many firms have positioned themselves as the service sovereign of their industry. Others have focused on the timeliness or efficiency of their particular offerings. Others have concentrated on convenience. Airlines and hotels have offered incentives for their "heavy users," with frequent-flyer and preferred-guest programs. Banks have promoted easy access to loans and flexible terms (within regulations).

The major growth in the hotel, banking, and airlines industries has occurred as a result of acquisition or vertical integration. The 1985-86 years witnessed unprecedented activity in airline acquisitions. Hotels, on the other hand, experienced significant growth through franchising and development. The Hilton and Marriott chains are excellent examples of this principle.

The strategy of growth through building and acquisition worked well for the major players in the hospital business in the early to mid-1980s. Whether based on the experience of the hospitality industry or merely on a lack of creativity, the large chains grew more formidable by increasing the size of their operations. Fortunately, much of the growth came through acquisition rather than construction. (Can you imagine 8,500 hospitals in this country?) The bottom fell out of this strategy in 1985, when utilization declines were experienced by the industry under DRGs and when some for-profit chains reported their first (ever) decline in earnings.

Marriott and other hotel chains have grown not only by additional units, however. As early as the 1970s, these firms were diversifying into other areas that appeared symbiotic with the core business. This practice is termed product-line or product-mix extension. Basically, it involves "extending" the product line into new areas not previously developed. The concept will be explored in detail in chapter 6, because it represents such a high degree of activity and opportunity for hospitals in the 1980s and 1990s.

Although there are many similarities among the service industries cited, there are myriad differences. Airlines do not have many product lines to offer. There are the various classes (first, coach) and there are distinguishable target markets (business, tourist, families), but the narrow "width" of the product mix (a firm's combined product offering) offers little opportunity for isolating specific segments of the business.

Hotels are, by and large, in the same predicament. Again, there are some differences in product offerings, (suites, double, single, studio), but the marketing efforts focus chiefly on the hotel name and the perception associated with it. It is our contention that hospitals actually have more in common with the consumer goods industry, which offers several products or services to a variety of market segments. Also, there are similarities with industrial firms, such as computer companies, that offer various lines to their clientele. We will draw on the lessons of those who have preceded us in order to avoid the pitfalls of pioneering.

References

1. Kotler, P. Strategic planning and marketing: defining their roles. Presentation before the American Hospital Association Society for Hospital Planning and Marketing, 1984 May 1.
2. Arthur Andersen & Co. and the American College of Hospital Administrators. *Health Care in the 1990's: Trends and Strategies*. Chicago: Arthur Andersen & Co. and ACHA, 1984.
3. Toffler, A. *Future Shock*. New York: Random House, 1970, pp. 139-44.
4. Touche Ross. *U.S. Hospitals: The Next Five Years*. New York City: Touche Ross, 1986.

Chapter 2

Marketing: The Switch Is On

"Greater than the tread of mighty armies is an idea whose time has come."

—Victor Hugo

Fortunately (for them), hospitals are not through changing. One of the painful, yet pivotal, changes is from a superficial to a sophisticated marketing mind-set.

The Road to Product Management

Advertising by Any Other Name...

When hospitals began to submerge themselves in the dark and threatening world of marketing, they moved cautiously but not comprehensively. Responding with the vehicle they knew best, the media, they altered course only slightly from public relations to advertising.

Everybody got into the advertising picture, unfortunately. A few advertisements were good, but most were poorly conceived and executed. There was the hospital that advertised "your hospital by the sea," in a coastal town where "even the view is therapeutic." Another ad featured a testimonial by a woman whose **late** husband never got the fine treatment anywhere that he got at Hospital X. But hospital administrators are quickly learning that the world will not beat a path to the door of the hospital that boasts a better lithotripter, even if that institution is warm and caring.

The initial flood of advertising has left a bitter taste in many administrators' mouths. The reasons are myriad, but here is a sampling:

- Advertising was done without sufficient preliminary research.
- The impact and results of advertising were difficult to measure.
- Advertising often irked physicians and, sometimes, consumers.
- There was a proliferation of "me-too," knee-jerk reaction advertising in response to competition. Misdirected messages meant confused consumers.
- There are only so many ways to say, "We care."

Savvy CEOs are recognizing that advertising is only a segment of a marketing orientation and occurs as the end result of a well-rounded strategic plan. In most businesses, advertising represents the finale, not the first act; hospitals have often reversed the order.

"Brave New World" Revisited

Now that health care professionals have had a chance to reflect and do some Monday-morning quarterbacking, the wise are going back to basics. From a marketing perspective, that means product management. And that's good for the industry.

Although product management is still a somewhat trendy buzzword that few understand and even fewer implement, the **switch** from "media madness" to marketing is happening. How do we know? This is evidenced through the following:

- More preliminary research is being conducted.
- Marketing plans are being written **before** the media plan.
- Advertising is beginning to focus on product lines, not on image campaigns.
- More marketing people within hospitals have true marketing backgrounds and are not just planners or public relations people.
- The literature, seminars, and consultants are talking product management.

Catalysts in the Equation That Leads to Product Management

A few of the variables that had an impact on the shift to a more sophisticated marketing mind-set are important to highlight. These

help substantiate the fact that the move to marketing is not fad-
dish but fundamental.

- **DRGs.** The models developed by Big Eight accounting firms
  are organized in product-line format. Although intended
  chiefly for cost control, the structure lends itself to a marketing data base and a blueprint for tracking results.
- **Consumerism.** "Consumer clout" over "provider prowess"
  is beginning to shake the bedrock of historical belief that the
  physician is the only customer worth worrying about. Some
  hospitals have patient advocates. Others are recruiting business people for their boards. Some are going so far as to offer
  money-back satisfaction guarantees.
- **Service orientation.** The "service supreme" sermons of
  Tom Peters, Ron Zemke, and others[1] strike a familiar chord
  with hospitals. The adaptation is comfortable, even natural,
  in an industry that prides itself on excellence of care.
- **Competition.** The free market brings out the best (and the
  worst) in everybody. There is nothing like competition to
  wake up sleeping dogs—or cash cows (products or services
  that have high profit margins), for that matter. As one
  administrator put it, "It's sink, swim, or get out of the pool."

Enter Marketing, Stage Right

All this is not to say that hospitals will teach hotels or airlines
something about marketing in the next six weeks. Far from it. The
progress is slow, but it is being made. As mentioned earlier, Kotler
suggests that the implementation of marketing in hospitals is
about 15 years behind the rest of industry, but that the gap will
close to 10 years by 1990. In actuality, the adaptation of marketing and product management principles is exponentially rapid
compared with other service industries. It has to be. The free
market has been thrust upon hospitals, and they have no choice.
"He who hesitates is not only lost, but miles beyond the next
exit," wrote one clever fellow.

The Benefits of Product Management

Small (and Segmented) Is Beautiful

The essence of product management is that the sum of the parts is
greater than the whole. Oversimplified, certainly, but particularly

apt in the hospital setting. In the absence of competition, not much attention need be paid to the parts as long as the whole prospers. In the presence of competition and the concomitant complexity, the winners will be those who can "think small," at least in product terms.

In his best-selling book *The Marketing Mode,* published in 1969,[2] Theodore Levitt urged us to think small in order to innovate, that is, create within the large organization the entrepreneurial equivalent of smallness. Similarly, in 1985, Gifford Pinchot III published a book titled *Intrapreneuring, or Why You Don't Have to Leave the Corporation to Become an Entrepreneur,*[3] in which he suggests that the alternative is stagnation and decline.

The immediate benefit of product management comes from focusing on the individual product or service segments and developing the strategies to enhance their volume and profit performance. The managers of the product lines become the "intrapreneurs," who look for new ways to differentiate and improve their service.

A parallel may be drawn to the historically pivotal battle of Sir Francis Drake against the Spanish Armada. In the present "battle," product management gives even the largest hospitals the ability to compete more like the smaller, swifter English fleet, rather than the larger and less maneuverable Spanish Armada. By breaking the whole into small, manageable parts and placing accountability squarely on the shoulders of the frontline managers, the entire organization benefits. Even the behemoths can become lean, mean fighting machines.

Product Management Focuses on the Bottom Line

Product management encourages innovation. The manageable size and financial focus complement competitive response. Competition fosters new products, services, and creative means to expand or enhance existing lines. Indeed, the effective product manager views the product line as his or her own business and champions its cause. One example of this was an administrative director for short-stay surgery at a hospital in the Northwest who became a product manager. He completed a detailed financial analysis of the operation that revealed a high portion of indirect costs more appropriately applied to the inpatient setting, not to outpatient surgery. He then successfully lobbied for a reallocation of those costs and immediately improved his bottom line. And lest you think that this reallocation was merely a shell game, let us point out that accurate costing will identify the true winners and losers in terms of the bottom line and will ultimately make those services more effective competitors. The sad truth of these times is that many hospitals have taken their "not-for-profit" subtitle too seriously. In fact, some have become "for-loss" hospitals.

Zeroing in on net income produces other important benefits: among them, well-defined accountability, consumer-specified research, increased focus on needs, and enhanced organizational efficiency.

Research Helps Determine Direction

Product management will result in a more targeted approach to providing services. This comes as an effect of the research and analysis that go into assessing the position of the product and the ensuing goals and objectives that are established. The research has a bias for action built into it; that is, it is designed to lead to results.

If we want to know what consumers think about our product, we ask them. Although this may seem self-evident, market research is still a relatively new tool in the hospital trade. But, given the penchant for numbers, market research may represent a valuable component in building a case for proposed strategies to accomplish hospital goals. The results of quantitatively valid studies cannot be dismissed by a subjective wave of the hand and should be readily accepted by board members and administrators as justification for whatever actions are implemented.

Under an organized product-line management function, market research is better targeted, more audience-appropriate, and easier to implement. The research can produce concrete conclusions that dictate practicable solutions, measured by follow-up research. For example, one hospital in Florida conducted focus-group research among the women in its community and found a basic dissatisfaction with the breadth of female services being offered. Based on these findings, the hospital developed a women's pavilion that addressed the needs identified through the research. The pavilion was an overnight success, in terms of both increased clientele and favorable publicity.

A Plan for All Seasons

The other major benefit to be derived from product-line management is increased effectiveness of the strategic plan. The long-range hospital plan encompasses all of the individual business-unit plans. Product management becomes the implementation phase for the grand plan on a small scale. This brings reality into the land of theory and thus makes the strategic plan more efficacious and pragmatic.

Although institutions have done an excellent job of long-range site planning and equipment-needs assessment, strategic planning is like a foreign language. But, as Arthur Andersen & Co. points out in its study *Health Care in the 1990s: Trends and Strategies,*[4] strategic planning will become the number-one issue among administrators. Product management facilitates strategic planning by focusing on strategic issues—what makes the product tick? Product management looks at the product line as a competitive entity. Strategies are then devised to develop a superior position vis-a-vis the competition. To borrow a favorite line from *The Art of War by Sun Tzu,* "All men can see the individual tactics necessary to conquer, but almost none can see the strategy out of which total victory is evolved."[5] The strategies in this case derive from a well-researched and well-analyzed situation. The tactic of advertising may be important to reach consumers, but the advertising is impotent if it does not address a specific product need.

The organization that adopts product management is also certain to improve its information systems and financial analysis capabilities. Product managers are continually asking, "Why?" and "Who is my target audience?" Traditional medical records and billing systems typically neglect key marketing information needs such as competitive pricing, source of patient origin, market share, and financial assessment by product rather than function. The advent of DRGs has helped to push hospitals to develop cost-accounting systems to address financial analysis concerns. The advent of marketing has added the need for further demographic and competitive analysis.

To summarize, the benefits of product management may be listed as follows:

- Better definition of each product/service segment
- A clearer view of the organization as differentiated from competitors
- A better understanding of how alternative strategies may affect the market
- Goals that are more action-oriented and meshed with organizational priorities
- A better understanding of the efforts that top management will need to take to achieve strategic objectives

- Improved implementation of plans and measurement of results
- Quicker response time to changes in the marketplace
- Better controls over costs
- A framework for financial decision making

The Environment Where Product Management Works

While it may seem to be a "blinding flash of the obvious," as Tom Peters and Nancy Austin term it in *A Passion for Excellence*,[6] competition is the key element that leads to the adoption of product management.

New Rules, New Players

When hospitals are faced with a declining census and an increasingly complex environment of regulation, alternative insurance plans, health maintenance organizations, primary care satellites, freestanding you-name-its, then product management flourishes. Under these conditions, product management affords a way of breaking up the entire hospital entity into its more manageable components.

In the absence of a fiercely competitive environment, product management still can be a boon to managing costs and profits under DRG reimbursement. But there is nothing like the fear of obliteration to stimulate creative management. Marketers (and product managers) thrive in a competitive situation where their talents are called on to achieve success in the marketplace. Trout and Ries, advertising executives and authors, term it "marketing warfare."

We maintain that the size of the organization is not as important as the commitment to a participative management style that involves several layers of administration in idea generating and decision making.

Some marketers may be resistant to product management because they fear a loss of power in a rigid hierarchy. One hospital marketing vice-president told us that she had already experienced the loss of one of her subordinates when she recommended setting up a product line for women's services, using one of the marketing staff as program manager. The hospital recognized only direct one-on-one reporting relationships and refused to recognize a dual functional and program management assignment. Thus, the marketer was assigned to report to an operational administrator.

This example is not uncharacteristic of many institutions that remain tied to a production mentality. Indeed, some of the more rigid organizations are seen in religious institutions, where a well-established hierarchical reporting relationship has existed for decades. The advent of competition may help to shake the traditional foundations and cause a soul-searching for new organizational approaches. It is out of this new thinking that product management can emerge.

Wanted: Progressive CEOs

It goes without saying that the support of the CEO is absolutely essential to the implementation of product management. That support needs to be evident in communicating the importance of marketing and product management throughout the organization and providing adequate funding to develop the organization and implement the resultant advertising and promotion programs.

The CEO is the ultimate product champion in supporting the marketing function. He or she can be educated in the principles of product management, but the support must be more than just lip service. That is, the CEO must continually reinforce the importance of the function in order to overcome enthusiastic apathy—an initial embrace followed by market inactivity. Our experience has shown that youth is a valuable asset in a CEO for understanding and accepting the marketing function. However, "youthfulness" is determined more by ability to adapt to new ideas and change than by mere age. Furthermore, there is still too much emphasis being placed on the attributes of administration and not enough on the rigors of strategic planning and marketing. The best administrators in the world cannot improve the condition of a terminally ill business if all they do is exercise their administrative abilities.

We always enjoy telling the story of how a CEO in the hospital business handed the new marketing director a copy of MacEachern's tome on hospital administration[7] (originally copyrighted in 1935) with all the reverence accorded to a copy of the Old Testament. After reading three chapters of the 1,316 pages, the marketing director tossed the book aside with the realization that things would never be that way again, that the age of competition would make the book's advice obsolete (if it has not already done so).

The Ally Within

Product management is grounded in the team approach. Although there is a team leader, there must be involvement from the several disciplines that support the product or service. In this case, marketing can act as the facilitator, but the operators must be involved in the strategy setting, decision making, and implementation. Indeed, the role of the marketer often becomes that of an educator in explaining how the process works.

Product management can be developed from within—it all depends on the flexibility of the individual to shift from an operations mentality to a volume, market-share, profit mentality. An organization that can think along entrepreneurial lines is a natural. Much has been written over the past year about the creation of "intrapreneurs" in the larger organizations. These small businessmen harbor the same beliefs as the product managers. One of the common elements that we've noticed in the many firms that have been surveyed in researching this book is the view of each service as a separate business.

Board support is also a key to success in implementing product management. If there are board members who understand marketing and have businesses of their own, seek them out to elicit their support.

It is also somewhat paradoxical that the threat of competition and an imminent census decline are stimuli to action that may be too short-term. It takes time to develop the product-management function within an organization and integrate it with the existing administration. Without the proper framework of organization and research to identify the leverage points, the whole process is doomed to failure. Take the time to set priorities and set realistic goals.

Conclusion

To conclude, product management will thrive best in an organizational setting that reflects and internalizes the ideas in books such as *Megatrends*[8] and is willing to embrace the marketing concept. Hospitals can survive through product management because it allows for a more detailed focus on the individual services as businesses, each of which must, as Ted Levitt puts it, "create and keep a customer."[9]

References

1. Zemke, R. *Service America.* Homewood, IL: Dow Jones-Irwin, 1985.
2. Levitt, T. *The Marketing Mode.* New York City: The Free Press, 1969.

3. Pinchot III, G. *Intrapreneuring, or Why You Don't Have to Leave the Corporation to Become an Entrepreneur.* New York City: Harper & Row, 1985.

4. Arthur Andersen & Co. and the American College of Hospital Administrators. *Health Care in the 1990s: Trends and Strategies.* Chicago: Arthur Andersen & Co. and ACHA, 1984.

5. Clavell, J. *The Art of War by Sun Tzu.* New York City: Delacorte Press, 1983, p. 28.

6. Peters, T., and Austin, N. *A Passion for Excellence.* New York City: Random House, 1985, p. 3.

7. MacEachern, M.T. *Hospital Organization and Management.* Berwyn, IL: Physician's Record Company, 1935.

8. Naisbitt, J. *Megatrends.* New York City: Warner Books, Inc., 1982.

9. Levitt, T. *The Marketing Imagination.* New York City: The Free Press, 1983.

Chapter 3

Product Management Review: The Industry Role Model

> "The general who wins a battle makes many calculations in his temple before the battle is fought. The general who loses a battle makes but few calculations beforehand. Thus do many calculations lead to victory and few calculations to defeat."
>
> —Sun Tzu

Product-line management was originally adopted in earnest in industry in the early 1960s as a way of managing the separate products or brands that constituted a company's multiple product offerings. The product manager's job was to manage the product through the various stages of the life cycle.

As was suggested in chapter 1, product management is less a vertical than a cross-organizational structure. The focal point of management is moved down through the organization to obtain more participative management. The product line itself becomes in essence a small company within the organization and functions as much as a separate entity as it does as part of the totality.

As product managers in industry, we used to think of ourselves as orchestra conductors. That is, we were responsible for bringing all the separate organizational functions together to work in harmony and create beautiful "music"—which was translated to sales and profits. We think the analogy is still apt, although the orchestra conductor has more real authority over the musicians than the product manager has over the various departments he or she works with.

Product management traces its roots to the early commercial entrepreneurs such as E. H. Stuart, who started the Carnation Company by selling evaporated milk himself door-to-door. He was the production man, salesman, market researcher, inventory manager, and advertiser all rolled into one. He was responsible for his own success or failure.

Similarly, product managers today identify with the success or failure of their respective products, even though they have much less authority over the operations than did the individual entrepreneur.

General Responsibilities of a Product Manager

A job description for a consumer goods company states that the product manager's general responsibilities are as follows:

> The product manager has responsibility for planning, developing, implementing, coordinating, controlling, evaluating, and adjusting comprehensive product programs that will ensure continuing product growth based on predetermined profit objectives. He or she acts as the focal point of all available departmental services, efforts, and planning necessary to achieve volume and profit objectives of assigned products.

Desirable Skills

To take this one step further, the general responsibilities of the product manager at this consumer goods company are reflected in a breakdown of 11 points that describe qualities and skills that are sought in the product manager:

- Ability to identify strongly and personally with the commercial success of the product, to understand its marketing problems, and to develop imaginative marketing plans for improving its position
- Judgment to define the relatively few important projects that will make the most significant contribution to the health of the product, and the subsequent discipline to concentrate on them
- Ability to get the most out of the many people who contribute to the planning of a marketing program
- Objectivity to forget "pride of authorship" once a program is initiated and to subject it to cold and painstaking review and appraisal against its contribution to the product's profitability
- Skills to use time and money in ways that will pay off the most
- Skills of a leader, an analyst, a diplomat, a salesperson, a coordinator, a fundamental management person, a self-reliant executive

- Ability to improve methods and techniques for organizing, planning, and controlling every phase of marketing activities
- Ability to play the part of coordinator in developing, evaluating, and implementing new products and product modification
- Ability to effectively use market research in product planning
- Ability to coordinate various plans with other company departments
- Ability to train and develop people under his or her supervision for more responsibilities

This list should be reviewed again when you are considering where you will find your own miracle workers to become your hospital product managers.

Major Functions

When asked to list the primary functions of a product manager in industry, we could enumerate them as follows, in descending order of importance:

1. Annual marketing plan
2. Advertising
3. Sales forecasting and budgeting
4. Sales promotion
5. Packaging and labeling
6. Test marketing
7. Pricing
8. New product development
9. Marketing research
10. Long-range planning

Although it is clear that the product manager in a hospital setting would have a somewhat different order of priorities and the jobs might not completely match (for example, packaging and labeling are of little importance in the service industries), the list serves as an excellent reference point.

Basic Management Activities

In managing the product line, the product manager performs five basic tasks:

- Assembles information

- Analyzes and evaluates
- Develops annual marketing or business plans and programs
- Presents recommendations to management
- Follows up on implementation

Let us examine each of these areas in more detail and relate them to the hospital industry, as they constitute the core of the product management concept.

Assembles Information

This encompasses both secondary and primary research:

- Historical volume, revenue, and profit trends: three- to five-year trends, along with a current projection.
- Industry and trade statistics: for hospitals the sources could be government—National Institutes of Health (NIH), Health and Human Services (HHS)—state health planning, hospital association, or university studies. Here we are looking especially for information on trends that affect the consumption or usage of the product line. For example, the acceptance of midwifery and the subsequent increase in nonhospital births will result in a decline in hospital births. Another, more relevant example is the increasing penetration of HMOs, because that growth could mean an immediate reduction in the total potential patient population. Age-specific disease rates are also the subject of study here.
- Demographic trend data: information on population trends (that is, 1970 versus 1980 census), along with projections for age groups and, by sex, birth statistics.
- Psychographics: the study of people's behavior and perceptions to the extent that such might influence a product. The sources of information are social studies, journal articles, and newspaper articles. The increasing interest in wellness and the life-style changes that can improve health would be considered here.
- Environmental changes: Regulation and reimbursement would be prime candidates for evaluation under this banner, along with the impact of alternative delivery systems. The shift to outpatient treatment and the concomitant improved reimbursement for outpatient procedures will accelerate the decline of inpatient utilization.
- Competitive data: market-share information, competitors' pricing, new product or service offerings. In the absence of a

regulatory environment that gathers such information, original market research may need to be conducted to obtain these data. It may be appropriate to visit competitors' facilities and watch what they do. Alternatively, one might talk to or visit noncompeting hospitals in other areas of the country to find out how their services may differ.

- Technology shifts: The continuing development of new technology has a direct bearing on the production efficiencies and capabilities of a particular product line. MRI will cannibalize a large portion of the computerized tomography (CT) business.
- Customer perceptions and usage: Original market research is often necessary to understand what physicians and patients think about your service and how it compares to that of your competitors. Patient surveys could be helpful here, but they don't provide a comparative benchmark to other facilities.

If this seems somewhat exhaustive, we assure you it is intentional. The more well informed a product manager is, the better will be his or her framework for decision making and strategy generation. Referring back to the quotation at the beginning of this chapter, the victorious product manager will be the one who assiduously gathers data and evaluates the situation prior to submitting a battle plan.

Analyzes and Evaluates

Having gathered all this pertinent information, the task is only half complete, because the product manager must then make sense out of it. The product manager must sift through the data and separate the proverbial wheat from the chaff.

This is a most difficult assignment for the budding product manager, because everything seems to be important. He or she must continually keep in mind the question "Is this going to have a real impact on the volume or profitability of my product line?"

Here the wise product manager will seek counsel from other, seasoned managers who can retain an objective viewpoint, who are not as close to the product and therefore can appproach the questions and data with a clarity of vision. In the case of hospitals, the product managers should utilize the marketing staff as a sounding board for ideas and conclusions reached in assessing the information at hand.

Develops Annual Marketing/Business Plans and Programs

The annual marketing plan is the cornerstone of any product-line building effort. The better part of three months could easily be expended in developing the initial plans for a product, which would then be updated and reviewed on a semiannual or annual basis. In industry, it is not uncommon to spend five months preparing a plan.

The process of getting people together in planning is essential to developing a working document in which all participants understand their respective roles. Commonly, the advertising agency is included in the process from strategic planning to simple development of copy and media sections of the plan. The marketing plan as a completed document becomes both an invaluable source of information and the marching orders for the coming year. Most plans have the same subdivisions:

- Internal and external background information
- Key findings reflecting data analysis
- Objectives
- Strategies
- Action plans
- Timetables
- Budgets

The plan itself is all-encompassing. That is, it delineates profit goals, pricing structure, product development, promotion, advertising, and so on.

There is no substitute for a well-structured, well-written plan. It forces people to focus on the important issues and supplies the framework against which results will be measured. Furthermore, it stimulates creativity by getting the product managers to think more about how they can have an impact, that is, what they can change or do that will significantly differentiate their product or service. **In short, development of the marketing or business plan is job number 1!**

Presents Recommendations to Management

The formal written plan is generally presented to management in conjunction with the budget request for the new fiscal year. The product manager has the responsibility for making the presentation to the upper management team, whose members generally represent several disciplines, such as marketing, finance, and operations.

The smart product manager will have presold major portions of the plan by seeking comments from the opinion leaders and respected members of the management team. If all components are brought into harmony prior to the formal presentation, the danger of surprises is minimized and expensive reworking is avoided.

Follows Up on Implementation

Once a plan is developed and approved by management, the job of implementation begins. The product manager has an immediate responsibility to ensure that all personnel who have anything to do with the success or failure of the product line are informed about the activities that are about to take place.

The plans themselves should identify the various tasks to be completed, the individuals who have responsibility for those actions, and the timing for completion of the tasks.

Again, as the orchestra leader, the product manager must ensure that the various functional departments are in harmony with the plan's objectives and are "playing" at the right time. The product manager must be unrelenting in following up the coordination of schedules and target dates.

The follow-up will also include regular reports to management on the progress that is being made in meeting plan objectives. Some product managers are permitted to make changes to meet varying conditions, without formal approval of the changes. Others, however, must obtain approval that varies from a casual to a strict, by-the-numbers format.

Characteristics of Product Managers

Product managers are entrepreneurial by nature. They want to make things happen—to do things differently and improve on the status quo. Many product managers selected their field of endeavor with the thought that it was as close as they could get to running their own business without actually doing it. Firms such as Procter & Gamble, General Foods, General Mills, Quaker Oaks, Heinz, and Lever Brothers attracted some of the best and brightest of the MBA graduates during the past 30 years. These men and women were fiercely competitive, with a drive to succeed and make their mark in the world of consumer packaged goods.

First and foremost, product managers were and are professional marketers who retain the customer focus over everything else. The degree of sophistication in marketing techniques varies by industry and according to the complexity of the product, but the focus, nevertheless, must be on the customer, for selfish reasons: if the product does not sell, the product managers cannot meet their volume targets.

Because product managers are generally responsible for a broad and diverse range of activities, they tend to be well organized and have the ability to digest large quantities of information while separating the important data from the unimportant.

Further, product managers tend to be iconoclasts who shun bureaucracy and administrative activities. Indeed, the innovative product manager is philosophically at odds with the good administrator. By definition, administrators are responsible for ensuring the smooth-running efficiency of an organization. However, if the goal is increased share, volume, or profit, something different must happen. Therefore, the product manager tends to ask the question, "Why do we do it this way?", in an attempt to develop alternative, more productive approaches.

Product managers devote full attention to their product lines. They are competitive and want to see their products succeed. This keeps them focused on the issues that affect their line to the exclusion of unrelated activities. This single-mindedness of purpose may be seen as a liability by some, but in truth it creates the intensive focus that is necessary to be innovative and productive.

Competitive but cooperative should be the refrain that is sounded here. Product managers must have the desire to be successful while recognizing that they need the cooperation of the rest of the organization to achieve a product's business objectives.

Product managers tend to change jobs frequently. In industry, it is unusual to find product managers with more than five years of tenure on a product. After three years, they get stale and need the challenge of a new product to stimulate their creative thinking. At the H. J. Heinz Company, product management was viewed very much as an up-and-out phenomenon. There were 10 product managers vying for two group-product-manager slots, whose normal longevity was twice that of the product manager position. Thus, there was considerable turnover in the ranks as the new assistants and associates earned their stripes.

Grading Performance: The Pass/Fail System

Although product managers may be evaluated on their ability to develop a good marketing plan, maintain cooperative relationships with other departments, and execute a well-conceived advertising plan, these subjective measures are clearly of secondary importance. Overall, product managers are rated on three criteria:

- Profit
- Sales
- Market share

The product managers' true objective is to achieve short- and long-term profit goals. They may do a superb job of building relationships with other departments, coming up with new product ideas, completing special projects, and so forth, but if they have not increased volume, share, or profit, the grade is "fail."

The goal-setting and performance-evaluation processes in the hospital industry are somewhat behind the times. There are too few institutions that have established a management-by-objectives (MBO) program that sets measurable objectives and identifies the individuals who have the responsibility for attaining those objectives. Indeed, the shift from performance standards based on multiple subjective measures to those based on the straightforward objective measures of profit, sales, and market share may be one of the most difficult transitions that hospital management makes. But, as difficult as it will be, the adoption of these measures will make a major difference in the mind-set of the managers.

When we first entered the business, we were told that one can do only two or three things well during a year. So why do we persist in setting 15 goals for an individual during a year? The simplicity of profit, sales, and market share is worth venerating.

Irreconcilable Differences between Industry and Hospitals

Product management in health care is more complex than it is in consumer products, industrial products, or even the other service industries. One of the most readily apparent differences is in the definition of "customer." In the packaged foods business, the consumer is the ultimate customer—period. However, in health care, we face multiple consumers in physicians, patients, employers, insurers, health maintenance organizations, and preferred provider organizations. Depending on what product or service we are discussing, distinctions need to be made as to what is important to each of these customers and how important each of the customers is in the purchase decision. Whereas the physician is still the main customer, the shift continues toward the patients making more of the decisions. In obstetrics (OB), for example, women are likely to select a physician who delivers at the hospital of their choice.

A second point of distinction is in the product itself. Although we speak of product lines, service lines might be a more accurate description. Furthermore, the services themselves may not be easily defined, as they may cross several disease and treatment modalities. For example, if you are looking at cancer care as a product line, you'll find that many of the DRGs have some cancer treatment components. In order to boil this down to a manageable entity, it may be appropriate to select only those DRGs in which 50 percent or more of the patients who are "true" cancer patients, that is, those whose primary disease is cancer-related, even though they may have several other complications.

The third major difference is that marketing in health care is significantly less sophisticated than it is in industry, and it is unlikely that the gap will be closed in the next 5 to 10 years. Marketing is often crowned as king in private industry, because it has a major impact on sales. The elements of marketing—promotion, packaging, and advertising—play a much greater role in industry. Indeed, a recent survey of Fortune 500 CEOs pointed out that 40 percent of them had marketing backgrounds. We know of very few marketers who are running hospitals. Marketing in health care is generally a longer-term proposition, inasmuch as people may go for years without using health services; there is relatively little opportunity to stimulate an impulse purchase for open-heart surgery. Therefore, the message must be consistent and sustained over time, with an eye to the future payoff.

The basic elements of the marketing mix—package, price, promotion, and place (distribution)—do not change from one industry to another. What does change is the emphasis that is placed on each of the individual elements. For hospitals, the emphasis shifts further according to the target audience. For example, patients have limited knowledge and ability to judge the actual quality of the technical services that are delivered in a hospital. That is why the compassion shown by the nursing staff and the quality of the food become important to them. Physicians, on the other hand, place more emphasis on the technical skills and equipment available within the institution.

The information that is currently available to consumer goods product managers is vastly superior to that which is available to hospitals. Firms such as A. C. Nielsen and Sales Area Marketing,

Inc. (SAMI) periodically report on product sales and inventories. This is in part a result of the length of time that marketing has been in place, but it is also a result of the necessity for measuring smaller changes. A one percent national share gain in beer or soap would mean millions of dollars to the company making that gain.

Finally, hospitals compete on a local or regional basis, in contrast to consumer or industrial products, which can be sold across the United States or even internationally. The product and marketing efforts for hospitals must therefore be tailored to the needs of the individual markets in which the hospitals compete. Although Humana may be attempting to establish a brand name for its hospitals across the United States, it will still need to compete on a localized basis in its product offerings. This thought is echoed by almost all of the major investor-owned and not-for-profit hospital systems and may be a strong counterforce arguing against the success of national networks such as Voluntary Hospitals of America (VHA).

Conclusion

Industry's experience and approach to product management provides an excellent backdrop against which to set the stage for product management in hospitals. At the same time, there are several distinct differences between the hospital and industrial setting that argue against an exact replication. Since marketing and competition are still relative newcomers to the health care field, the adoption of product management in hospitals will require a great deal of education and experimentation before a prototype approach becomes a reality. Nevertheless, although differences do exist, the industry role model is worthy of emulation in the separation of product lines as freestanding businesses with their focal point clearly on the needs of the customers.

Chapter 4

Finding the Miracle Worker: The Hospital Product Manager

"We are moving from the specialist who is soon obsolete to the generalist who can adapt."

—John Naisbitt

Finding a good product manager in a hospital setting is a little like finding a nongambler in Las Vegas. The problem is that most hospitals want to promote internal candidates (and perhaps rightly so), but historically the hospital environment neither encouraged nor rewarded the skills of a product manager.

Therefore, hospitals have started to recruit more product managers from the outside, usually from service or consumer goods industries. This creates a problem, because imported product managers are immediate strangers in a foreign land. They must try to assimilate the culture, learn the business, and introduce a new discipline all at the same time. Add to this the need to demonstrate remarkable results on a shoestring budget, and one can envision the dilemma. All things considered (and all things rarely are), we feel that the best plan is to find the product managers from inside. Because that is not always a possibility, we shall explore several options.

What to Look For

A product manager should be a combination of Lee Iacocca, Alexander Haig, Henry Kissinger, and Rodney Dangerfield.

The product manager needs to champion the product or service for which he or she is responsible. In so doing, the "persona" of that product will become identified with the attitude and enthusiasm of the manager. As with Iacocca, the chairman of Chrysler Corporation, the success or failure of the line may have a strong correlation with the manager's ability to represent its cause and be its spokesperson. Iacocca personified the spirit of Chrysler (feisty, hardworking, and uncompromising) to a believing public. In many ways, the product manager personifies a product line to its "customers."

Like the former secretary of state, Alexander Haig, the product manager must have the attitude of "I'm in charge here" (as Haig incorrectly stated after President Reagan was shot), even if it is not true. If the product manager is not assigned or does not assume direct responsibility for the product, no one will. Assignments without accountability usually fall short of the mark. Persons willing to put their careers on the (bottom) line, depending on the success or failure of the service, may prove to be a rare species in a hospital setting. That is one reason why good product managers tend to be mavericks with an entrepreneurial spirit.

The product manager must be a diplomat. Like Henry Kissinger, the esteemed negotiator, product managers should move easily and comfortably in many circles. They will need to discuss policy with hospital administrators, pursue detail with technicians, and mingle with the medical staff. Most important, the product managers must converse with the consumer. In fact, public perception is really the first language in which a good product manager must be fluent.

Finally, the product manager needs to have a sense of humor. Like Rodney Dangerfield, it is likely that the product manager "won't get no respect" (or will get less than deserved) from many of the traditionalists in the organization. To counter this, the product manager must be somewhat self-deprecating and possess the ability to laugh at the follies of bureaucracy.

Of course, no one assumes that the product manager will develop these rare talents in short order. It may take a month or two, or even a year. During that training period, the marketing vice-president and perhaps the CEO will need to provide helpful support and encouragement.

Where to Look

Theoretically, the best product managers should come from industries or companies where product-line management has become a science. Consumer goods companies such as Procter & Gamble, General Mills, Quaker Oats, or Heinz would arguably be the best training ground. These companies understand consumers and how strategic business units (SBUs) can most effectively be segmented to target the most appropriate markets and maximize the bottom line. However, their type of person may find the complex structure of hospital protocol somewhat compromising and encumbering and may also be uncomfortable with smaller advertising and promotion budgets and a general lack of awareness and respect for the marketing function. The consumer goods professionals come from an environment where marketing is king and enter a setting where marketing is a fling, or so some think.

Nonetheless, if the hospital is in a highly competitive position, if the board is business-oriented, the physicians are progressive, and the CEO is market-driven and possesses a thick skin, these marketing professionals "will make it happen," and few do it better.

Another group to tap is the service marketing professionals. In a 1986 study by Garofolo, Curtis & Company,[1] a sample of 50 marketing professionals rated this group as the most likely group "from which to hire a hospital marketer," if one were hiring from outside the organization. The service marketers have worked in industries where the dynamics closely parallel those of the hospital. Many service industry marketing managers know what working with a small marketing budget is like, because that is all they have ever known. They are accustomed to smaller staffs, less sophisticated advertising, and fellow workers who are baffled by the marketing role in their business.

The industries that make the best training ground for service marketers are banking, hospitality, and hotels. These are the areas mentioned most often for service industries in the study by Garofolo, Curtis & Company. As noted in chapter 1, these specialties, as well as their marketing specialists, can offer great insights into previously proven techniques.

Criteria for Decisions

Each hospital will need to decide which industry would constitute the best training ground for product managers. Here are a few general guidelines to consider in making the choice:

- Board member orientation
- Nature of the bureaucratic model of hospital

- Individuals within the hospital with similar experience
- Salary and benefits parity with industries
- Upward mobility for professionals
- Level of tolerance at all levels for new ideas
- Time frames to get programs up and running

As highlighted in other chapters, consumer goods marketers are not proving to be good long-term candidates. Service marketers seem to be working out better in terms of fit and length of tenure. However, if the hospital is willing to take a risk, why not call on a good old consumer goods manager who has a track record for selling soap and who should thus be able to market cardiology, as well.

External Imports

There are, of course, pros and cons to hiring people from the outside to do the work of the product manager. We'll discuss both, based on the trends we've seen.

Square Pegs

The major drawback seems to be the problem of "fit." As mentioned in earlier chapters, the world of packaged goods is drastically different from that of a hospital, and when a product manager from the packaged goods industry (or even the service industries, to a lesser extent) enters the corridors of the hospitals, both parties have their guard up. Hospitals are understandably conservative and move much more slowly than the "risk it and ride 'em" pace of industrial marketing. As stated in chapter 3, product managers are entrepreneurial and somewhat iconoclastic. Naturally, that type of personality struggles inside a hospital setting.

Too often, from the administration's viewpoint, there is a shrouded picture of marketing as a necessary evil, a concept to be tolerated but not embraced. This may manifest itself more in the purview of the marketing director than that of the product managers, but the latter will sense the vibrations throughout the organization and, unless they are prepared adequately to deal with the phenomenon, the resistance may prove too unwieldly.

There is also a major barrier to empathic entry that few marketing types are prepared to deal with—the physician component. The marketer in business is accustomed to dealing directly with the consumer or through sales representatives who take their marching orders from the consumer.

Understandably, the first response of the imported marketer is to bypass the traditional "gatekeeper" and reach out for the end user of hospital services. The harsh reality is that, even though times are changing and consumers are taking a more active role in health care decision making, the doctor still controls the entry and exit parameters of the marketplace. To ignore doctors in that process is a *faux pas* that far too many hospital marketers have committed. As a result, the credibility and viability of the science of marketing have come into question, and some administrators have abandoned its application as too risky, despite the potential returns.

Of course, many of these problems can be alleviated if the vice-president of marketing or the CEO helps to facilitate the product manager's assimilation into the organization. In that regard, the product manager may undergo a scrutiny that is uncomfortable and uncharacteristic of the profession. Nonetheless, the new kid on the bureaucratic block cannot be expected to grasp a system and a structure that is unique in and unto itself without some assistance.

We would suggest, therefore, that new employees in marketing be given clear guidelines as to what they should and should not expect. Otherwise, the organization will find itself in a position similar to that of the hospital in the Midwest that hired four product managers from Procter & Gamble, only to lose them one year later because of functional frustration. Product managers are trained to manage for results, but the truth of health care administration is that results alone do not a hero make. Rather, how the results are achieved plays as important a part as the outcome itself.

For a Few Dollars More

Another very real problem in hiring from the outside is dollars and cents. Because product managers are usually on a fast track, they expect to be compensated well for their time. Even though the best marketers at companies such as General Mills, Carnation, or Colgate-Palmolive do not achieve the stratospheric salaries of MBAs pursuing consulting or investment banking careers, their stipends exceed those of most middle managers in hospitals. In some cases, the salaries exceed even those of higher-level managers. The study of 50 hospital marketers, by Garofolo, Curtis & Company, found an average annual salary of $38,000 for those with a bachelor's degree and $52,000 for those with a master's.[2] (It should be noted that the ranges varied significantly by region.) We are told by health care marketing experts that one should expect to pay between $40,000 and $50,000 for a product manager with one to three years of experience. So the marketing director may have to pay a rather lofty salary in order to attract a manager that is industry-trained.

Even the base-salary issue does not stand on its own. Most product managers in industry are on some form of incentive system. Those hospitals that have implemented a bonus or profit-sharing system have found it quite effective, but there is major resistance to the concept, especially among the not-for-profit hospitals. There may also be internal resistance because of the perceived inequity of such a system. Nonetheless, the administration must deal with the reality that good product managers are operating on a motivation mechanism that involves an incentive for bottom-line performance.

We would suggest a system that ties incentive reimbursement to performance through the product-line teams. In this fashion, the rewards are spread more evenly and everyone (theoretically) has the opportunity of reaping the benefits of an effective product-line structure. In order to do this, the objectives of the product line must be clearly stated at the outset and the measures set in place for evaluating the achievement of stated goals. These, then, can be reviewed periodically (as will be mentioned later) so that realistic expectations for remuneration can be established. Rewards as simple as a congratulatory dinner for the triumphant product management team may be sufficient to start the process and satisfy recognition needs at the beginning. As the system evolves, however, a more tangible and substantive incentive should be incorporated into the results mechanism.

Here Today, Gone Tomorrow

The final concern with hiring external professionals to fill the product management function has been referenced indirectly. Qualified professional marketers are quite mobile. They have qualifications as generalists that are unusual in the health care field. Consequently, the risk of high turnover (and reduced organizational loyalty) is a bona fide consideration. As mentioned earlier, the managers from Procter & Gamble lasted less than a year. A good friend of ours who had been hired from General Mills became frustrated with the glacial pace of health care marketing. She left a top job with a major midwestern hospital after less than two years.

Another Procter & Gamble veteran left a position as vice-president of a health care consulting firm after three years to start his own operation. The list goes on and on.

Those marketing vice-presidents or CEOs expecting loyalty and longevity, then, should face reality and realize that such would be the exception rather than the rule. Empirical evidence would seem to indicate that abbreviated tenure is the order of the day. Administration should count on a one- to three-year horizon for external marketing professionals. That is the case in the industrial and service industries, and to expect otherwise in the hospital setting is unrealistic.

Arguments For

Why, then, given all these obstacles, hire from outside the hospital setting? There are basically four reasons.

First, marketing is not a science, art, or discipline (label at your own peril) that is easily acquired by the untrained observer in an abbreviated training period. Marketing is as much a mind-set as it is a mechanism. However, for most, it requires some battleground experience to be fully appreciated and assimilated. This usually cannot happen vicariously through the case-study method or through a shortened learning curve that forces participants to learn while they earn.

Therefore, if there is no one in the organization who understands the marketing mode, internal candidates are unlikely to comprehend it in a time frame that will produce meaningful results. Most hospitals do not have the luxury to wade through the muddy marketing mistakes that would probably result under improper training or tutelage.

The second reason deals with the competitive mentality. Most hospital professionals are just beginning to incorporate terms such as **competition, market share,** and **return on investment** into their vocabulary. It may take another few years before they internalize the philosophy underlying such jargon. Hence, the need to respond to marketplace pressures may be met with the kind of paralysis through analysis that often accompanies a regulated industry. The professional marketer brings a sense of urgency, yet maintains market savvy to resist the reactive responses that have characterized competitive challenges over the past three years.

Moreover, the entire organization will probably benefit from the perspective this one individual brings to the organization in terms of a well-thought-out approach to the forces that are fragmenting the hospital's resources and threatening to undermine its viability as an operating entity.

Third, along that same vein, the professional marketer is valuable for the fresh viewpoint he or she brings to the industry and the institution. Although no one person is an island of ideas, a new look at old ways is often incentive enough to hire someone not strapped into traditional approaches. One of the first things an outsider will do is challenge the way things are done. This is especially true of MBA-trained product managers, who spend one to two years in an atmosphere of Socratic skepticism, challenging anything that appears in a case study.

This critique by brash (and often young) newcomers can be abrasive and cause considerable defensiveness if the administration and staff are not prepared to handle such "unique" actions. However, the behavior can be beneficial if accepted for what it is. This, then, becomes one of the truly valuable advantages to hiring a professional marketer, whose provocative perspective may either paralyze or propel.

Finally, the trained marketer brings an element of change to the organization. By bringing someone from another industry and another philosophy into the hospital, a clear message is transmitted. A philosophical commitment in the form of an individual conveys that message much better than memos or seminars. Much has been written about "change masters," but we would propose the need for a "change champion" who personifies the evolution from bureaucracy to business, from regulatory to anticipatory actions. No other functionary better qualifies as a change champion than a professional marketer. It is his or her business to constantly assess the changing needs of the marketplace in order to marshal resources to satisfy those needs.

Pros and Cons of Hiring Outsiders

In summary then, the pitfalls and possibilities for hiring outside product managers are listed below:

Pitfalls
- Forced fit between product manager and hospital
- Administration's view of marketing as a necessary evil; atmosphere of apprehension
- Outsider's misunderstanding of the physician role
- Salary expectations high, incentives required

- High mobility means rapid turnover, reduced loyalty

Possibilities
- Already knows a function not easily learned or assimilated
- Brings a sense of competitive urgency and appropriate response
- Personifies the organization's willingness to change
- Brings a fresh perspective and provides a new look at traditional methods

Inspired Insiders

Just as there are pros and cons for external candidates, there is a similar dichotomy for internal product managers.

Arguments Against

Many of the reasons for not hiring from the inside are elaborated in the section on external candidates. The challenge of understanding and implementing the marketing mind-set may be too much to expect for a staff member who has been (for most of his or her professional life) more concerned with service than share, or with relations rather than return. Several studies indicate that Americans have the attitude that health care is a right, not a privilege, and that every American is entitled to it. Many health care professionals share that sentiment (if not champion it), and it is therefore very difficult to shift into a competitive mode that necessitates winners and losers as dictated by the market. This basic philosophy, then, can prove the undoing of some health care professionals as product managers.

Another fundamental flaw in trying to convert insiders into product-line managers is the problem of specialist versus generalist. Health care is primarily a specialist field. This has generated a mind-set that everything needs to be neatly structured and understood from a historical perspective. The American Medical Association rarely makes a move without years of research that support its recommendations. Hospital administration tends to mirror that attitude. This means that hospital staff members who are assigned the responsibility of product management may struggle with the nebulous nature of the assignment and the need for proceeding into uncharted waters.

Another major concern that confronts inside converts is what we term the "detail detour." The nature of health care professionals is to be focused on detail. That is altogether natural and expected in an industry where human life is on the line and the details matter very much. However, too many managers can become entrapped by the detail and become ineffective in implementation. This is not to say that marketing programs do not require research and homework to back up the action portion of the plan. However, there comes a time when the big picture must be viewed. This is sometimes a difficult task for health care professionals and needs to be a major consideration in the selection of the product manager.

One final con to hiring from the inside deals with the health care professional's proclivity toward conservatism. There is an inherent risk in the marketing function. The organization must consider people who are willing to assume that risk; otherwise, the organization will always be playing catch-up with the innovators and "me, too" will be the modus operandi. In today's competitive environment, such a strategy will not keep an organization afloat for long.

Arguments For

In our minds, there are more positive reasons for hiring from the inside than there are reasons against.

The first and foremost reason is actually the converse of the rationale mentioned early in the discussion of hiring outsiders. Marketing is already a foreign language, with a certain amount of built-in resistance. If the language and the process can be softened with a familiar face and juxtapositioned jargon, the message may more likely be accepted and the programs implemented.

We saw this phenomenon firsthand when an internal marketing manager suggested a program that had previously been denied and shelved. Once the well-known, well-respected line manager presented the program, the idea was heartily welcomed and the money readily allocated. Such has also been the experience of several of our colleagues.

Another good reason for hiring from within is the system itself. An inside promotion will result in a manager who is familiar with the hospital and with its political structure. Most important, the health care pro will understand the dynamics of the physician component and will be prepared to deal with physicians as the key constituency. Also, the doctors will be more easily disposed to dealing with the product manager when it comes to mapping out the mutual objectives that affect both the hospital and its staff. Again, an example from our experience illustrates this point. A program met resistance from a group of doctors when presented by a person they did not know or trust. However, the same program was accepted when formatted by a "coworker" (hospital staff member) with whom they were familiar.

The health care professional also knows the industry and may have a good sense for what is missing in its ranks. Whereas the outsider may bring fresh perspective, the inside candidate may be more realistic in an assessment of what needs to happen to change the organization's position. There exists within many organizations the type of people who take the macro view, even though their responsibilities may not require such perspective. They are the type who read *The Wall Street Journal* on their lunch hour, though it is not directly related to their job. If that kind of person is attuned to the needs of the industry, he or she will make an ideal candidate.

Another valuable reason for hiring insiders is that it sends a message to the staff that the organization is willing to develop its own people in making the marketing transition. Although this may sound somewhat circuitous based on the "change champion" idea proposed earlier, the same argument applies, only on a different level. By hiring from outside, the administration is indirectly positioning itself as internally unable to adapt to the challenges and changes being thrust upon the industry and its players. By keeping the opportunities inside, the organization is, in essence, saying, "There are great possibilities in this hospital as we move into this exciting new dimension of health care management." Thus, the organization is more likely to adopt the principle of product-line management at all levels.

Pros and Cons of Promoting Insiders

In summary, then, the reasons for and against promoting product managers from within are listed below:

Pitfalls
- Lack of a competitive mind-set
- Specialist mentality may not work with generalist necessity
- May get bogged down in detail and miss the big picture
- Idea of risk and innovation may be too foreign

Possibilities
- More likely to be accepted
- Understands the system

- Understands the industry; proposals may be more realistic and applicable
- Sends message for internal opportunity
- Organization more likely to adopt principle through heightened sense of ownership

Conclusion

The decision to hire product managers from inside or outside depends on each hospital's unique situation. For the most part, we recommend hiring the majority of product managers from inside, because they, and therefore the concept, will have a better chance of being accepted. But wherever the new managers come from, the most critical factor in their eventual success will be the respect and support they get from key administrative and medical personnel.

References
1. Farrell, L. *1986 Annual Hospital Marketing Professional Survey.* Ardmore, PA: Garofolo, Curtis & Company, 1986, p. 13.
2. Farrell, L., p. 4.

Chapter 5

Defining the Product Lines

"There is no such thing as a commodity. All goods and services can be differentiated and usually are."

—Ted Levitt

DRGs Provide a Framework

The initial interest in product lines began roughly in 1983, with the CPA firms' investigations into case mix management alternatives under the prospective payment system. The accountants were convinced that hospitals would need to have a clear definition of their products and the costs that go along with those products. On this basis, much of the early literature and experimentation with product lines centered around accurate cost analysis.

The aggregation of closely related DRGs to constitute various product lines is most appropriate from a financial and data management standpoint. Inasmuch as the medical information systems are now structured on DRGs, it is only natural to use DRGs in composite as the product line. Further, the advent of cost-accounting systems will permit relatively clear assessment of the revenues, costs, and profits for each of the DRGs. This cost-accounting information is rapidly becoming indispensable, because the ancillary services make up such major parts of the products/services.

Although many hospital administrators may look back fondly on the pre-DRG days, in truth, the advent of DRGs has heightened the interest in product lines or strategic business units and has provided the framework for product-line definition. Still far from perfect, the DRGs have established a consistent measure across all hospitals that facilitates comparison and analysis.

Through the Eyes of the Marketplace

The definition of product lines based on cost is easy for hospitals to comprehend, inasmuch as this reflects the traditional cost-reimbursement Medicare system. However, **true product lines have their focus on the marketplace,** not on operations or production. We cannot emphasize this enough. The countryside is "littered with the bones" of those individuals who have strayed from the path of customer orientation. Patients just want to get their hearts fixed and get back home. They do not care that you have echocardiology, a catheterization laboratory, and so on. One does not market hospitals or physicians—one markets services. Although it is true that as hospitals we serve a multiple-client list of doctors, patients, employers, and insurers, what we offer to these diverse groups is service.

As a starting point, the accounting firm Ernst & Whinney detailed several criteria for identifying product lines; they called them strategic program units.[1] These criteria are useful reference points as we begin the process of defining product lines, and they warrant further scrutiny. It would be a mistake to try to isolate any one of these criteria to the exclusion of the others. Their value lies in establishing groups that are identifiable and manageable as separate businesses within the hospital.

Ernst & Whinney Criteria

- Be identifiable to the market
- Have an identifiable market
- Contribute significantly to hospital long-range planning and daily operations
- Be an identifiable diagnostic category
- Have unique or dedicated production facilities, staff, and technology
- Be recognized as a unique or special program
- Be an administratively manageable unit
- Have linkage to treatment patterns of medical staff
- Parallel the organization of the medical staff

It should be noted that Ernst & Whinney begins its list with "Be identifiable to the market" and "Have an identifiable market." By adopting these criteria, we immediately rule out nursing services, radiology, lab, pharmacy, social workers, and other ancillary support services. We also eliminate specific procedures unless we are dealing with the specialized needs of one of our customers. For example, it would be logical to think of the hospital as providing heart services. Under heart services, we would include open-heart surgery, electrocardiograms (EKGs), echocardiograms, percutaneous transluminal coronary angioplasty (PTCAs), cardiac rehabilitation, and cardiac catheterization. Open-heart surgery would not be a line itself but might be broken out as a major component if we were negotiating a package price for an HMO or an insurer.

Definitional Considerations

Early attempts to use the 23 medical diagnostic categories (MDCs), which are groups of DRGs, as product lines have proved unsatisfactory. The MDCs are simply too broad and not sufficiently well defined for market purposes.

Indeed, the DRGs themselves are often less than satisfactory in defining a product category. There is no way around this problem, and adequate time must be given to ensure that the correct DRGs are being used. For example, when we were first looking at neonatal intensive care as a product-line subset of maternal and child health services, it was discovered that two of the DRGs classed as neonatal intensive care units (NICUs)—#389 and #390—had only 15 percent and 5 percent actual NICU cases incorporated in them. We determined this by sampling medical records. As a result, revenues, costs, and profits for the NICU line were altered significantly from the original projections.

Perhaps the most complex product-line definition problem is encountered in the cancer product line. When we first tried to assign DRGs to the cancer line, we discovered that there were 184 DRGs (39 percent of the total 470 DRGs) that had some element of cancer diagnosis and treatment associated with them. The solution to this problem was again discovered in actually scrutinizing patient records. In order to constitute a reasonable base to measure for market and financial purposes, a committee reviewed the DRGs and determined that only those DRGs with 50 percent or more cancer patients would be included in the cancer product line. Thus, the cancer line was reduced to 46 inpatient DRGs and 1 outpatient DRG (representing radiation oncology).

Identification Eases Management

Above all, the product lines need to be identifiable to the hospital and medical staff so that their management can be facilitated. Obviously, the more definite they are, the easier this task becomes. Emergency services is an easily definable entity that can be managed as a product line, as contrasted to cancer services, which encompasses radiation therapy, surgery, chemotherapy, and numerous nursing service support components.

Attempts have been made to define product lines as specific nursing units. Although this has been a traditional way of tracking patients and provides a good base of historical formation, it may work for only a limited number of products. For example, most mental health patients are isolated in a mental health nursing unit, but there may be other mentally ill patients in the hospital who have a physical problem that separates them from the mental health unit. There needs to be some accommodation that allows their inclusion in the statistics.

Let Users Help

The utilizing public itself may also define product lines for you. For example, if an HMO wants to contract with your hospital for obstetric services, it may be entirely logical to manage obstetric services as a separate product line. What we need to address is the question of substance: Does the service generate enough revenue to be managed as a separate entity? The ability to package and market birthing services directly to the public has facilitated making obstetrics and related services the first true product line for many hospitals. The scope of those services has recently been expanded into the idea of women's centers, where a variety of women's services such as mammography, ultrasound, osteoporosis screening, health information, and education are provided in addition to obstetrics and gynecology.

Is It Worth Worrying about?

When Ernst & Whinney comments that a product line should contribute significantly to hospital long-range planning and daily operations, this means that the line must generate enough revenues to be of concern. That is, if your hospital grosses $75 million in annual revenues, why pay any attention to a product/service that generates $40,000 in annual revenues? We would have trouble arguing that a product line that brings in less than one percent of total hospital revenues would be seriously worth considering. It is easy to spend as much administrative and mental manpower against a small service as against a large service, with the ultimate payoff being low for the small service. This lesson of priority setting is often lost on administrators who become overly enthusiastic in the pursuit of the small picture. A more systematic approach needs to be employed; this is discussed in chapter 11, Reviewing the Results.

Other Approaches

Ernst & Whinney does not bother to suggest which of the criteria are most important nor whether you can establish a product line if it does not meet all the criteria. This is not to say that we are critical of their approach. They have offered us an excellent starting point from which to proceed in making our own judgments. In the interest of contrast, let us take a look at some of the other approaches to product-line definition that have been attempted.

Humana's Centers of Excellence

Although neither Humana nor any of the other hospital management companies has yet to fully implement a product management system, the "Centers of Excellence" approach that Humana adopted in 1982 is reflective of what product management can accomplish in differentiating a service. Although the Humana program is not an attempt to define product lines, the segregation of special services for reasons of investment funding, promotion, or physician recruiting is worth emulating as a way to get started in experimenting with the product management approaches to strategic management organization.

Humana's definition of a Center of Excellence, as guided by Dr. David Rollo, senior vice-president of medical affairs, and Dr. Thomas Moore, vice-president of medical affairs, is as follows:

> A Center of Excellence is a referral and consultation center that provides the highest quality of care in a given clinical specialty in a geographic area.[2]

The center has three essential elements represented in a triumvirate—hospital, physician group, and medical education and clinical research program—as illustrated below:

	Hospital	
Physician group		Medical education and clinical research program

These elements are necessary to achieve recognition by corporate headquarters as a true Center of Excellence. Within each of these three elements, certain criteria have to be met in order to pass the first hurdle of consideration:

- **Hospital**
  - —Has an established reputation for excellence (as demonstrated in community and physician surveys)
  - —Has complete diagnostic and therapeutic support services that feature state-of-the-art technology
  - —Has a nursing staff competent in the clinical specialty that earns it professional recognition
  - —Has an administrative staff that effectively integrates the Center of Excellence into overall hospital operations
- **Physician group**
  - —Has exceptional diagnostic and treatment skills in its specialty
  - —Practices state-of-the-art medicine and remains current with changing technology and methods through its participation in education and research
  - —Has professional knowledge and skills clearly recognized by peers
  - —Has stable and effective leadership
  - —Has productive professional relationships with primary care physicians, peers in its specialty, and the faculty of a medical school
- **Medical education and clinical research program**
  - —Has defined medical education and clinical research plans
  - —Is directed and controlled by an advisory board
  - —Provides for a productive relationship with medical schools

The benefits to the institution that met the screening criteria and then successfully passed the evaluation phase to become a full-fledged Center of Excellence included infusions of capital from the Humana corporation, as well as funds from the Humana Foundation for education and research ($100,000-plus), and special recognition within the Humana organization. As of the end of 1986, there were 23 centers throughout the 90-hospital system. Among those, there are 11 separate specialty areas: cardiovascular (5), diabetes (5), orthopedics (3), women's (2), neuroscience (2), ophthalmology, pulmonary, spinal injury, urology, gastroenterology, and burn.

The objective behind the centers—to create something unique and different that will stand out among the competition—is also a prime objective of product and marketing management. To the extent that Humana is segregating a service and managing it as a unique property, it is creating a product line within its system.

Branding, Texas Style

Republic Health Corporation in Dallas has taken a different approach in "branding" its services, which are consumer-responsive and can be marketed throughout their system or to other systems. As of this writing, Republic has identified 10 "product lines," as follows:

- Gift of Sight—cataract surgery
- Step Lively—podiatric services
- You're Becoming—cosmetic surgery
- Call Me—alcoholism treatment
- Sound Sense—hearing exams
- Impotency Solutions—urology service
- View—women's health problems
- Miracle Moments—obstetrics
- ReNew—cocaine addiction treatment
- Reach—adolescent psychiatric treatment

Republic refers to these programs as a branded products strategy. Brand management is generally focused on the advertising that is necessary to establish name recognition with the customers. At Procter & Gamble, the persons who supervise brand managers are even given the title of advertising manager. The product manager, on the other hand, is more of a generalist who is concerned with packaging, product, technology, distribution, and inventory management, along with advertising and promotion. Although this distinction between brands and products may seem a bit academic or pedantic, it is relevant to the distinction between what Republic is doing and true product management within hospitals. Republic has developed a communications-centered advertising and promotion package for specific services. What they have not done is develop a system for managing product lines.

Brand vs. Program vs. Product-Line Management

A good deal of confusion still exists over what product-line management really is from a definitional, as well as a practical execution, standpoint. Most of the hospitals that we have contacted personally or about which we have read portray what we define as "program management." The following comparison is included to suggest an increasingly comprehensive approach to organizational management in moving from brand management to product-line management.

- **Brand management** is the least intensive of the three, with a primary focus on advertising and promotion, for example, Adventist's "Ask a Nurse" program, Humana's "Instacare" program for emergency services, and Healthwest's "ElderMed."
- **Program management** brings an added dimension of focus on the service components that make up the program area, but the advertising and promotion elements are still dominant. Program management tends to limit itself to a few select programs in the hospital, which are often segregated out as warranting special attention. Health Corporation of America (HCA) is pressing ahead with exploration into programs in geriatrics, women's health, and occupational medicine. The NKC, Inc. has program managers for their women's pavilion, spine center, and geriatric services (see chapter 12, Case Studies).
- **Product-line management** presents the most comprehensive approach in its complete management of separate business entities. The ideal is to organize the entire institution, not just a few selected program areas, under the product-line management approach. Decision making and responsibilities are pushed downward through the organization as top management becomes more strategically oriented. The product team will assess all the cost or purchase elements, establish budgets, conduct research, and measure results. Goals are reflective of the financial as well as the market orientation and shy away from traditional administrative duties. Nurses may be reassigned from the general nursing staff to a particular product area such as rehabilitation or same-day surgery.

Conclusion

To conclude, the definition of product lines still requires some experimentation but appears to be moving closer to groupings that are recognizable to the patient population. The identification of specific diagnoses that make up the product line will be an essential part of the historical data analysis and future results-tracking mechanisms.

Finally, as a practical matter, some product lines will receive little initial attention, even though they represent a major source of revenue in the institution. General surgery and general medicine are two such examples. Although it is convenient to identify these catchall groupings as product lines, there is little that can be done to effectively change the market dynamics of these lines.

At the very least, when setting priorities, we must keep in mind that it is best to devote administrative and management efforts to those lines where there is the greatest potential for increasing volume and share, as well as to take advantage of emerging trends. This would normally rule out general medicine and general surgery as top-rank candidates and would instead focus on areas such as maternal and child care, emergency care, outpatient surgery, elderly services, and mental health services.

References
1. Ernst & Whinney. *Strategic Program Unit Planning: Strategies and Management Tools for a Product-Oriented Marketplace.* Chicago: Ernst & Whinney, 1983.
2. Moore, T., M.D., vice-president of medical affairs, Humana. Personal communication, December, 1986.

Chapter 6

Extended Product Lines: Variations on the Theme

"The reasonable man adapts himself to the world; the unreasonable one persists in trying to adapt the world to himself. Therefore, all progress depends on the unreasonable man."

—George Bernard Shaw

In June 1986, *Health Industry Today* featured an article entitled "Extended Product Line: Preparing for the Consumer Revolution in Healthcare."[1] Written by the journal's editor, David Cassak, the article discussed an important innovation in health care—extended product lines (EPLs). Work on this new idea was spawned in Minneapolis by Peat, Marwick, Mitchell and Company and InterHealth. The concept of EPL was to look beyond the traditional services perspective of the hospital and to broaden it to a consumer perspective based on the episode or case. That is, EPL looks further than the three traditional delivery components—hospital, doctor, and outpatient services—to the rationale for an entire continuum of care. It explores things such as consumer financial concerns, education, dietary and nutritional needs, housekeeping, psychosocial services, and so on. In many ways, the approach is similar to the concepts of holistic medicine, which treats the patient as an entire human being rather than just addressing the symptomatic disease or injury.

The Value of EPLs

The real value of EPL exists in opening up people's thinking and reorienting a focus on the consumer. A successful implementation of the EPL concept could lead to locking up the referral stream that results in inpatient stays. It recognizes that a patient has

53

many needs beyond the simple delivery of a hospital service and, in meeting those other needs as well, the hospital becomes a bona fide "full-service" provider. If a consumer attends education classes, receives financial counseling, and gets nutritional assistance at your hospital, that familiarity through contact should lead to usage when the occasion arises.

EPL can also lead to vertical integration strategies. In order to lock in the potential patient from cradle to grave, the hospital adds the other services that are naturally tied to the episode. Financial counseling might be a good example. In obstetrics, the InterHealth hospitals discovered that people had many concerns about finances other than simply those related to who would pay for the delivery and hospital stay. These other considerations may well have an impact on whether the family decides to have a baby in the first place. By providing financial counseling, the hospital (or, more appropriately, the health care system) will be filling a customer need that bears a direct relationship to the provision of health care services.

EPL is not significantly different from a true product management system but is substantially different from mere program management that is promotion-oriented. A good product manager should be thinking about ways to provide a more encompassing service in order to enhance revenues and maximize usage of the core service.

Industry as a Model

The concept of extended product lines is, of course, not new to U.S. business. Marketing professionals in various industries have tried it for years. In the packaged goods industry, the idea has spawned many worthwhile products or lines of products. The fundamental thrust of the concept is slightly different, however, in the industrial setting from what is currently being discussed by Cassak and others. In industry, the extended line usually applies to products or services within the same basic realm of operation.

Product Line versus Product Mix

As hospitals view the idea of extended product lines, they might be well advised to align their approach with this orientation, while recognizing at the same time that what are being touted as extensions of the product line are really diversifications into new territory. Even though some marketers are quick to point out that the hospital's basic mission should guide the exploration and development of "extended" services, a critical point of differentiation lies in this basic understanding of the product-line process.

A case in point: When General Motors decided it was going to start offering its own financing mechanism some years back, this could hardly be construed as an extension of any of its current product lines. This represented an entirely new business for General Motors—in essence an extension of the firm's product mix.

Similarly, if a hospital decides that it will begin offering financial counseling prior to a couple's birthing experience, the service may or may not fit into the obstetrics product line. Most likely it does not. It is not a service that most hospitals offer in any shape or form, and the consumer perception of a hospital offering that service may inhibit ready acceptance it. Most hospitals' exposure to financial counseling is confined to dealing with people who cannot pay their bills. The service is offered subsequent to customer interface, not precedent to delivery of the service. Hence, would-be parents may initially resist a hospital service that offers "financial advice" that extends beyond method of payment or basic pricing information.

Aside from the issue of perceptual conflict, there remains a larger concern with viability vis-à-vis the competition. Why, for example, should the hospital be able to market a line of children's clothes (T-shirts) better than a national manufacturer or even the local garment houses? Aside from first-time contact with the end user, what does the hospital have to offer? Certainly not the buyers' expectation of the service.

The Elusive Concept

Finally and most critically, this type of EPL may detract and deter managers from the basic operations of effective product-line management. Empirical research seems to demonstrate that the concept (of product extension) is not easily grasped, let alone implemented, at the hospital level. By introducing this "revolutionary" way of approaching the idea, the management of the hospital may find itself charting a new course in a very foggy environment. Consequently, the goals outlined by the principles of product management may fall short of the mark while attempting to be conceptually avant garde. The words of a former college professor come to mind: "You can't understand Greek until you've mastered English."

A Traditional EPL Approach

We do not want to convey the idea that we are opposed to the concept of product-line extensions. On the contrary, as we have mentioned elsewhere, the premise is a fundamental one to ensure a successful long-term implementation of product-line management.

What the health care professional needs to understand is the basic difference between extending the product line and entering a new business (extension of the product mix). What we are talking about is much more than semantics. The differences are pivotal to the basic understanding of the entire function of the product-line manager and staff members who assist with the planning and implementation of strategies.

Definition

We would define an extension of the product line, as it relates to hospitals, as any service or product that programmatically and perceptually falls within the realm of the basic services offered by that product line. A cardiology product-line manager who decides to extend the product line by adding cardiac rehabilitation services meets little philosophical or programmatical resistance. However, if the same product manager opens up a heart-healthy restaurant, he or she has entered unfamiliar territory with minimal expertise. That is not to say that such expansions will not or do not work. The point is that such a broadly defined "extension" goes beyond the scope of the product manager and his or her committee, in most instances, and may be contrary to the image that the customer has regarding hospital service. More important, it drains off resources from the basic product and, although it may result in some incremental revenues, it may divert attention from more lucrative ventures associated with the core product.

Guidelines

We would therefore recommend the following guidelines in evaluating services for EPL:

- Does it fit "comfortably" within customer perceptions of the product line? A case in point: When Fisher Price developed a tape recorder to follow on the heels of its successful phonograph, no one was surprised. In fact, it was expected and greeted with greatest welcome by the buyers of the phonograph.

- Does the product-line staff or manager have the resources to pull off the project with minimal reallocation of resources?
- Does the existing administrative staff have the managerial background and skills that relate to the new product or service? For example, operating a catering service out of the hospital food service department requires a different set of skills from those involved in serving a captive audience on the hospital site.
- Do the incremental profits achieved by the extension exceed the opportunity costs (in this case, as measured by additional profits from focusing more attention on existing products or services)?
- Do the extensions meet the basic "mission" of the product line? If not, do such extensions offer opportunity for redefining that mission while maintaining the integrity of the overall organizational mission?
- Does the hospital offer a differential advantage over current competition that justifies development of the concept?
- What impact will offering the service or product have on existing customers or clientele (such as third-party payers, physicians, and employers) and established business patterns?
- Would this service be better handled as a product-mix extension with an entirely different cast of characters and a different mind-set and approach?

Examples of Product-Line Extensions

One hospital with which we are acquainted decided to offer radiation therapy as part of its overall cancer line. In our minds, this represented traditional product-line extension. It rounded out the existing product line and was an addition expected by patients and physicians alike. The service did not detract from existing business; in fact, it made a valuable contribution in terms of increasing the overall demand for the full line.

Another case in point is the home health agency that began offering nonnursing services, such as homemaking, cooking, reading, and general around-the-house services. This type of service represented a good fit because the general perception of such services was already there. In fact, many people are surprised to find that home health nurses do not offer those services as a natural extension of their activities in visiting people's homes.

Conclusion

The concept of extending the product line is not new. It has been around as long as the existence of product-line management. However, the approach to EPL should closely align itself with the existing or proposed product-line management system. It is valuable to differentiate between what we have defined as product-mix extension and what we are calling product-line extension. This distinction is important because it reflects the degree of understanding and subsequently the probability of successful implementation of the product-line management concept.

Some hospitals have made EPL an art, while others have made new-venture development their hallmark. Every hospital needs to incorporate both areas of expertise if it is to survive into the 1990s.

Reference

1. Cassak, D. Extended product line: Preparing for the consumer revolution in health care. *Health Industry Today.* 1986 Jun. 49(6):13-25.

Chapter 7

Developing a Marketing Data Base

"The more extensive a man's knowledge of what has been done, the greater will be his power of knowing what to do."

—Disraeli

One of the biggest disappointments of seasoned marketers upon first entering the health care field is the paucity of data that permit assessment of a hospital's marketing position. Historically, records have been kept and maintained for medical and billing purposes, not for financial or marketing purposes.

In consumer goods industries, people are used to having at their fingertips on a monthly basis data that details volume, share, and profitability for the products in question. There are also data available on where the consumers live, their ages, sex, income, and other demographics. Alas, when we first started to work with hospitals, we found that this type of information was generally not obtainable or at best was available on a one-shot basis and thus did not permit any comparison of trends. Although many of the data elements were collected in the process of completing medical records, the data on those records were not entered into the management information system (MIS).

Further, reporting systems have traditionally focused on inpatients with little data gathered on ambulatory visits. Again, this means that we are limited in our ability to develop any historical pictures for those outpatient product lines.

There is hope in the changing environment. Within the next five years, the information gap should be closed. The advent of uniform billing codes, DRGs, and other standard reporting requirements will help to ensure consistency and comparability of information. Employers, HMOs, and insurance companies will also speed us along to better-quality data that track their memberships' utilization of a particular institution.

The more widespread use of personal computers will permit us the flexibility to analyze and massage the data once we have obtained them. Existing mainframe systems are simply not flexible enough to meet marketing needs. The MIS support staff currently focuses on payroll, billing, accounting, and medical records, often to the exclusion of market-based information. We're reminded of the old Woody Allen joke: "There is a fate worse than death... Have you ever spent an evening with an insurance salesman?" We might substitute "day" and "management information specialist" for "evening" and "insurance salesman" without losing the message.

The Basic Necessities

In the pursuit of knowledge that will permit the development of sound conclusions regarding health care product lines, there are certain basic bits of information that must be obtained. These are:

- Volume data—discharges or visits, patient days
- Patient origin—zip codes
- Patient demographics—age and sex
- Market share
- Competitive pricing
- Financial data—revenues, expenses, net income
- Major admitters
- Payer mix

Let us next examine each of these information pieces separately to understand what sources we can look to in gathering the information and why it is important. In the preparation of product-line business plans, we recommend looking at three-year historical trends (we'd prefer five-year but realize that the data are probably not available or, if available, are inaccurate) on all the basic necessities.

Volume Data

Discharges and patient days are basics that do not need much discussion. The DRGs making up a particular product line are aggregated, and the average length-of-stay figures are calculated. We should emphasize that discharges and not admissions are the key measure, as the ultimate reason for a patient's hospitalization may differ significantly from the admitting diagnosis.

On the outpatient side, patient days and discharges are not applicable. Visits and workload units are more appropriate measures of volume. At the time of this writing, several outpatient services are still considered exempt units that do not require reporting under DRG formats. Thus, a separate reporting system needs to be created for these units.

Patient Origin

In order to target your services/products most effectively in the future, it is imperative to understand where your patients are coming from. Zip codes provide the base information and can be aggregated into service-area markets, that is, metro areas, counties, and so forth. Zip-code data are preferable to census tract information. Census tracts are much smaller, thus adding to complexity in assessment, as well as being relatively useless from a communications standpoint. That is, you can direct mail to selected zip codes but not to census tracts. Therefore, it is often appropriate to assign census tracts or portions thereof to zip codes.

Some state hospital associations and state health planning organizations are now gathering patient zip-code information. Oregon, for example, through the Oregon Hospital Association is gathering data on patients from all hospitals in the state. This information is then collated and reformatted to identify each hospital's share of discharges by zip code.

Once you have obtained the zip-code data for the product lines, each line can be compared against the others to see what the relative importance of the line is in that particular geographic area.

Patient Demographics

Patient demographics can be useful in identifying differences and unique characteristics of a product line for purposes of market development. Age and sex are the most salient demographics worth gathering with regularity. Medicare has helped in this regard by segregating the population above age 65. However, the growing elderly population above age 65 demands further refinement to separate the youthful aged (65 to 74) from the older (75-plus) age group.

As an example, if you were to look closely at the patient profile of mental health admissions, you might discover that two-thirds of the patients are women and two-thirds are between the ages of 14 and 39. If advertising is developed to support the mental health program, it should then feature women in that age group.

Market Share

Market-share data are basic to an understanding of whether you are winning or losing in the marketplace. In consumer products, this data could be obtained regularly from private firms such as A. C. Nielsen, which actually measure shelf space allotted to products in supermarkets. Unfortunately, we do not have the ability to "measure," or count, patients in hospitals without upsetting the nursing or administrative staffs. Therefore, we must rely on other ways to obtain this information.

Some states, such as Washington, have a reporting requirement to develop the comparative data. In the absence of any organized authority gathering the information, this must be done through market research—consumer attitude and usage studies that ask, "Were you or any member of your family hospitalized during the past year and, if so, where?" or other intelligence-gathering methods.

Competitive Pricing

Pricing of specific services is taking on more meaning with increased competition and contracting arrangements. Until a few years ago, prices for hospital services were dictated by cost or expense and target margins, not by the marketplace. Product management's approach is to use pricing as one weapon in the competitive arsenal to gain market share, along with the other elements of advertising, promotion, product differentiation, packaging, and so on.

In contrast to volume, origin, and demographic data, which are obtained through hospital reporting mechanisms, prices must generally be obtained from other sources. Rate increases filed with state agencies are useful but do not specify enough detail on individual services.

One way to gather pricing data is through the "market basket" approach. In this approach, 10 of the most common procedures that make up a product line are specified and then other hospitals are surveyed for what they charge for those procedures/services. The data are then indexed against your hospital to determine what the variations are. Table 2 shows a comparison among three hospitals of seven prevalent short-stay surgery procedures. In this

Table 2.   Pricing Comparison of Selected Short-Stay Surgical Procedures

	Hospital A		Hospital B		Hospital C	
Procedure	Price	Index	Price	Index	Price	Index
Cataract with lens implant	$850	100	$1,200	141	$1,050	123
Myringotomy	200	100	350	175	210	105
Dilation and curettage	250	100	500	200	390	156
Laparoscopy	350	100	400	114	475	136
Hernia	400	100	400	100	450	113
Arthroscopy	600	100	500	83	750	125
Breast biopsy	350	100	300	86	250	71

case, hospital A is indexed at 100 and the other hospitals are indexed in comparison. For example, hospital B's index of 141 for cataract surgery with lens implant is calculated by dividing $1,200 into $850 times 100. In quick translation, this means hospital B is 41 percent more expensive than A for cataracts. As we scan the example, it is apparent that, with few exceptions, A has a pricing advantage over B and C.

A further refinement of this technique is the application of weighting factors to each procedure to develop a weighted average comparison, as shown for hospital A in table 3. For example, cataract surgery was performed 10 times for each myringotomy during a specified time period; therefore a "10" value was assigned to cataracts and a "1" value to myringotomies. The price times the factor was then multiplied to get a weighted extension. Having done this for each procedure, the weighted extensions were then totalled and divided by the total of the weighting factors for a composite average price of $530 for hospital A.

Financial Data

In running any business, be it investor-owned or not-for-profit, we need to understand what our revenues, expenses, and net incomes are to properly allocate resources of the institution. In evaluating product lines in hospitals, we often need to create a new cost-accounting system to accurately portray the finances of a particular line. Historically, financial statements have centered around nursing units and functional service departments.

Although the nursing unit may have come close to describing the product, there was generally little attempt to allocate the other

Table 3.   Weighted Average Pricing Comparison for Hospital A

Procedure	(a) Price	(b) Weighting Factors	(a × b) Weighted Extension
Cataract	$850	10	8,500
Myringotomy	200	1	200
Dilation and curettage	250	5	1,250
Laparoscopy	350	3	1,050
Hernia	400	4	1,600
Arthroscopy	600	2	1,200
Breast biopsy	350	3	1,050
Total		28	14,850 ÷ 28 = $530

functional services to that unit. For example, the mental health nursing unit may have isolated the service fairly well, but there was no allocation of pharmacy charges and expenses to that unit. Therefore, the profit picture varied substantially when the two were combined.

In order to obtain a clear view of the product line, a detailed cost-accounting system is required. Through the use of a micro-computer, one can step down the costs for each department and assign them to a particular DRG. The combination of the DRGs then paints the total financial picture. Most larger hospitals (those with 250 or more beds) either have adopted or are in the process of adopting a cost-accounting system that will satisfy the needs of product management. The only trick is getting the financial data to interface with the marketing data. But, then, that's probably grist for several chapters or another book.

Major Admitters

Keeping your customers happy is axiomatic in every industry; health care is no exception. Because physicians are still the number-1 customer of a hospital, it makes sense to know which ones are most important to your success and contribute the most profitable patients. An understanding of this emanates from a ranking of physician admissions for the DRGs that compose the product line. At a minimum, you should develop a list of the top 25 doctors, ranked by admissions, with an indication of the percentage of total admissions for which each of those physicians accounts. This will tell you at a quick glance whom you need to keep happy.

Payer Mix

All hospitals have been tracking Medicare and Medicaid patients as separate from those with standard insurance. However, with the growth in alternative delivery systems, it has now become important to refine payers further into HMOs, PPOs, self-pays, welfare, or charity. Also, you might want to take a look at the major employers to ascertain how important they are in admissions to the hospital.

Standardizing the Process

In implementing a product management system in any institution, it helps to have a standardized set of forms or formats on which to gather or present the data on a product line. By going to a standard format, there is a consistency and readability among all the business plans. For example, figure 1 shows a sample format for reporting data on patient admissions, patient days, and average length of stay, and figure 2 depicts a typical financial reporting format for a not-for-profit institution.

For further amplification, figure 3 presents a fill-in-the-blanks format, developed for a Louisiana hospital, that is effective as a means of educating department managers about what needs to be addressed in order to have a complete understanding of their product line. Although some clarification of the questions would no doubt be required by the managers, the questions themselves should be enough to stimulate the creative juices while demonstrating that this is not a task to be addressed with casual attention.

Product Fact Book

When you really get organized, you can put together a product-line fact book that contains a plethora of information related to each product line. In consumer goods, we used to refer to the fact book as our bible, because it contained the wisdom of all that had transpired on that product over its lifetime. In these days of high turnover among personnel, we recommend it highly as a link to the past that facilitates ready understanding of what has been tried, what has worked, and what has failed. Besides the basic marketing data described here, it may contain market research, product budgets, competitive profiles, advertising copy, promotion data, seasonal indexes, and price increase history.

Figure 1. Sample Format for Reporting Patient Admissions Data

Trends in Admissions, Patient Days, and Length of Stay

Years _____

Year	Patient Admissions	Patient Days	Annual % Change in Patient Days	Average Length of Stay
_____	_____	_____	_____	_____
_____	_____	_____	_____	_____
_____	_____	_____	_____	_____

Figure 2. Sample Format for Reporting Financial Data for a Not-for-Profit Institution

Financial Statements
Years _____

	Year 1	Year 2	Year 3
Gross revenue less deductions	_____	_____	_____
Net operating revenue			
Operating expense Direct Indirect	_____	_____	_____
Total			
Excess of revenue over expense	_____	_____	_____
As percent of gross revenue	%	%	%

Figure 3. Product Analysis Sheet

I.   PRODUCT DESCRIPTION
    1. Name and describe product_____
    2. Manager of product_____
    3. Delivery location_____

II. PRODUCTIVITY MEASUREMENT
    1. Definition of product unit_____
    2. Revenue per unit_____
    3. Cost per unit_____4. Profit (loss) per unit_____
    5. Number of units per day/week/month___6. Profit per day/week/month_____

III. TARGET MARKET
    1. To whom sold?_____
    2. Who makes decision to purchase?_____
    3. Sex_____Age_____Health condition_____
    4. Is health condition recognized?_____
    5. Income level or other financial considerations/ability to pay_____
    6. Other health considerations/limitations_____
    7. What is size of population needing this product (give source of data)?_____
    8. Where do patients come from geographically?_____
    9. What market "niche" does this product fill?_____
    10. What does this target market already know about us in relation to this product?_____
    11. Upon what basis does this target group decide to buy this service?_____
    12. Where does this target market get its health information on this subject?_____

IV. SERVICE DELIVERY AND PACKAGING
    1. How will clients access the product?_____
    2. Is it convenient?_____
    3. How will they pay for it?_____
    4. What is time cost and other costs to client?_____
    5. How will they locate product in the service unit and overall hospital?_____
    6. How will other hospital personnel respond when asked about the product?_____
    7. What provisions are made for their comfort while here?_____
    8. What educational materials are provided?_____
    9. What follow-up, support groups, aftercare are provided?_____
    10. What is traffic flow in the department?_____
    11. How will you monitor waiting time?_____
    12. What gimmicks or goodies are used as giveaways?_____
    13. How are staff, physicians, residents trained to deliver service?_____
    14. What special touches would enhance delivery of product?_____
    15. Are there fluctuations in service delivery? Distribution trends?_____
    16. Where is technology headed?_____
    17. What is expected rate of growth (give source)?_____

V.   STAFFING
    1. Position_____
    2. Education, training, or level of expertise_____
    3. Hours_____4. Salary_____

Figure 3. **Product Analysis Sheet (continued)**

VI. MEETING THE REGS
     1. Licensing required_____
     2. Federal, state, city laws_____
     3. JCAH requirements_____
     4. Insurance required_____
     5. Malpractice needed_____
     6. What are trends in the regulatory area?_____

VII. EXISTING/FUTURE COMPETITION (make copies for each competitor)
     1. Pricing_____
     2. Strengths_____
     3. Weaknesses_____
     4. Position among all competitors_____
     5. Budget_____
     6. How clients are being obtained_____
     7. Future competition expected_____
     8. Description of how product is marketed_____
     9. How do you stack up against the competition for this product?_____

VIII. PROMOTION/SELLING STRATEGIES
     1. Personnel needed_____
     2. Sales materials_____
     3. Publicity_____
     4. Advertising_____
     5. Personal sales calls_____
     6. Sales goals_____
     7. Other_____

IX. MONITORING PRODUCT SUCCESS
     1. What data are needed to measure cost effectiveness?_____
     2. Who gathers these data?_____
     3. How will you measure client satisfaction? Who measures it?_____
     4. How are growth patterns monitored?_____
     5. Other service ideas_____
     6. Research needed_____

X. SPIN-OFF BENEFITS
     1. Image-building for hospital_____
     2. Cross-selling of other products_____

XI. OTHER STUFF
     1. Is there an alternate source of funding available?_____
     2. What gut feeling/intuition do you have that cannot be qualified?_____
     3. What specific growth is possible for this product?_____

Reprinted, with permission, from H. Gary Allen, Lakeside Hospital, Metairie, LA.

Chapter 8

Setting Up the Management Team

"What the business enterprise needs is a principle of management that will give full scope to individual strength and responsibility and at the same time give common direction of vision and effort, establish team work, and harmonize the goals of the individual with the common welfare."

—Peter Drucker

Unlike the situation in manufacturing and service industries, hospital marketers are not surrounded by functional managers who willingly and cognizantly support the core effort. Rather, marketing personnel must do considerable hand-holding through the early stages of implementation, hence the need for formalizing a supportive structure that facilitates the product-line management process.

That structure must be initiated by the CEO, who must send clear signals through appointments, assignments, or restructuring that the support is consistent throughout the organization. "We're in this for the long haul" must be the resounding message sent and understood. St. Luke's Medical Center in Phoenix was one of the early experimenters with product management. As far back as 1972, it assigned management personnel specific responsibility for program areas such as orthopedics, cardiology, ophthalmology, and behavioral health. The product managers at St. Luke's were responsible for cutting across functional service areas to ensure that the needs of the primary customers—doctors—were being met.

St. Luke's went through several changes in management and revised the approach to product administration in the early 1980s when they hired fresh MHA candidates and tried to make them product managers. Inasmuch as the MHAs lacked experience and a marketing focus, they tended to gravitate toward administrative management and empire building, to the exclusion of a strategic

69

marketing approach. The resultant dissatisfaction with this product management approach led to its demise in 1985.

Among the lessons learned by the St. Luke's experiment was the conclusion that the matrix organizational approach is very difficult for people to adapt to and that the pursuit of the product management concept over time bears a direct relationship to the CEO's commitment to the process. When a new CEO came on board who had little vested interest in the concept, it quickly faded into obscurity.

This chapter describes a model currently in use by hospitals throughout the country in establishing the product-line management team.

Product-Line Committees

Under this format, a group of people sit on a committee to decide and determine direction for the product line. The committee (or team) can consist of either technical members of the various disciplines involved in the line or staff members from various functions contributing to the line, or both.

For example, a committee overseeing the efforts of the cardiology product line might involve the following:

- Administrative director, cardiology
- Medical director, cardiology
- Supervisor, outpatient diagnostic facility
- Nursing director, intensive care unit
- Finance manager
- Administrative director, radiology
- Lab supervisor
- Director, surgical operations
- Assistant administrator
- Marketing manager

The group might meet monthly to discuss marketing strategies and, most important, to address the action phases of the business plan. The cooperation of the various members is most critical around the budget period, for that is the time that needs the most extensive interaction and coordination.

This group is very much a proactive one and should view itself more as a venture team than as a board of directors. The committee should take collective responsibility (and be given collective accountability) for the achievements as outlined in the business plan.

To the extent that the hospital offers monetary reimbursement and visible recognition, the group will assume an increased level of responsibility in its role as primary influencer of hospital policy and procedure for that particular line. Although anathema five years ago, many hospitals are experimenting with profit incentives or bonuses to these groups, based on bottom-line performance. Our experience in industry indicates that such financial incentives are practically necessary to guarantee continued success of this approach.

Along with this, the teams or committees should have a competitive thrust internally. Pitting the product-line management teams against each other in measuring impact on revenues and income can have a positive effect on overall morale and heighten the sense of service urgency. In this regard, middle management will be beating down the stodgy barriers of bureaucracy and, as a result, the entire hospital will benefit.

Organizing for Success

To get the process started, there needs to be a high level of visibility. The CEO should inaugurate the first product team and perhaps even attend a few of the meetings to get the feel of the system. This practice will also convey the message that the process is of great value to the organization. Internal publications or newsletters should run an article or two on the committee, and even a presentation at middle-management staff meetings would be appropriate.

The first committee should involve team players who are effective collectively and who will pull off a success. In this regard, it is better not to have too many representatives from one function (say, three nurses), because they might unite (and not cooperate) if things don't go their way. One hospital got off to a very slow start when four members of the committee decided they did not like the committee chairman.

Because the chairman is so vital in leading the group, consideration should be given to making the committee head an assistant administrator or a high-level department head. The responsibility for leading the group does not have to rest with the product manager, although the structure should eventually move in that direction.

Even if an assistant administrator or a vice-president is not directly represented on the committee, he or she should maintain active involvement through regular reports or updates. These should also be forwarded to the CEO or administrator.

Detailed minutes of the meetings should be kept so that the

group can keep an internal check on its progress, as well as allow for future groups to mimic or modify the original team.

Most important, the success of the entire group, rather than individual achievement, should be stressed. The product manager will be held accountable for the bottom-line results. If the manager is sharing that responsibility with an entire group, there is likely to be greater cooperation when it comes time to marshal the resources to achieve the defined objectives. This is especially true if the objectives have a group consensus.

Molehills out of Mountains

The group should be given realistic expectations and should set realistic objectives. There may be a tendency for the team to reach for the moon to prove itself a local hero. In reality, however, unattainable goals are to everyone's disadvantage. This is where the marketing professional or the business-savvy vice-president needs to perform a reality check. Many health care professionals are accustomed to preparing forecasts and projections based on full-time equivalent (FTE) need, not on market reality. There must be a realist in the group who can identify optimal, yet reachable, objectives.

To this extent, the administration should select a product line with a high probability for success. This concept will be discussed further in chapter 10.

The Task at Hand: A Business Plan

The first task of the product-line team should be to draft a business plan. This is especially true in a matrix line such as cardiology or oncology. A matrix line is defined as one whose services or products cut across several functions. Although the committee should not physically write the plan (document by committee has not been successfully performed since the King James version of the Bible), members of the group should be instrumental in gathering data and providing direction for future strategies and forecasts.

It is the job of the product manager (with help from the marketing department) to draft the business plan. Hence, we have another good reason for a top executive to chair the committee. The executive will have more success in receiving the data and forecasts required to put the plan together.

Development of the business plan is no easy task, as we hope you will better appreciate after reviewing the materials required to complete one. Therefore, a realistic time frame should be allowed for the first draft. We suggest two to three months, depending on the sophistication of your current information systems and the availability of competitive analysis. The first plan may take a full six months to develop, but discouragement should not supersede the necessity of putting the plan into place.

Once the plan has been approved, with modifications from the executive staff, all available resources should be channeled toward achieving the goals and objectives outlined therein.

Marketing's Role

Assuming the organization has decided to launch the concept with internally promoted line managers, the role of marketing is more that of coach/counsel/colleague. Under this system, it is important that those staff members in the marketing department give the line managers enough basic understanding of the process so as not to frustrate them in their early attempts. The marketing staff are basically facilitators in the process. Because they are the recognized professionals in the function, they must provide enough support so that the operations staff members (now marketing converts) will experience success in their first marketing efforts.

The more the process can be streamlined with forms and standardized formats, the greater the probability for a positive experience and a successful outcome. As mentioned in earlier chapters, the jargon of market share, incremental volume, and marginal costing are "Greek" to these new product managers. To expect them now to set realistic and responsible goals in these areas is presumptuous but may be feasible if assisted by someone who has been there before.

To that extent, the marketing director or vice-president and his or her staff cannot expect a few classes or seminars on marketing management or product-line implementation to bring the product managers to a level of cognizance that will produce worthwhile business plans. Most product-line structures we have witnessed have a marketing staff member on the product-line committee. Although this is a necessary start, it is not sufficient on its own. The marketing director needs to assume full responsibility for assisting the product managers in their function, even if they have operations reporting relationships.

In some hospitals, the marketing department contains all the product managers. Under this scenario, the reporting steward-ship and accountability factors are well defined. In those organizations where the product managers continue to report through the operations function, the lines of authority can get a little muddied. Hence, there is a need for a clear understanding of functional accountability and assistance.

Inasmuch as the drafting of the business plan is one of the product-line committee's (or the individual product-line manager's) first and most important responsibilities, we reiterate the recommendation for standardization. The more it can be formatted in a "cookbook" style with a fill-in-the-blanks mode, the more smoothly the process will flow. This is especially true for a hospital that is trying to implement several product lines at one time. For those organizations that are experimenting with one or two, there is room for more creativity and uniqueness, but there is still the basic need to make the planning process as efficient as possible. As mentioned earlier, this may argue for hiring a product manager, with prior business planning experience from outside the organization. However, it can be a great learning opportunity for several staff members, as they work their way through their first business plan.

In essence, the business planning experience can be fabulous or it can be a fiasco. The outcome will depend largely on the "front" work that the experts in marketing initiate.

What To Do in the Absence of a Marketing Staff

What do you do if your organization does not have a marketing professional to act as tutor? Do not assume that the newly converted product manager can draft the business plan by osmosis or that the product-line committee can work it out "if given enough time." That is a fatal mistake, and one too often repeated by organizations that should know better.

One course of action is to hire a consultant to walk the committee, task force, or product manager through the process. If there is a committee, the relationship of that consultant can be as an adjunct member of the group. By hiring a consultant (and there are several who specialize in the drafting of business plans), the organization can establish a precedent for the first plan and formalize a system with a proven performer. In so doing, the hospital will have saved itself the potentially onerous task of trying to redo or undo an ineffective plan.

Another option for developing the first business plan is to bring in someone on a part-time basis. This person, working on retainer, becomes an integral part of the planning process but does not cost the hospital a full-time salary with benefits. We know hospitals that have worked with university professors, professional marketers, and entrepreneurs who have gone on to form their own businesses but still have time to develop a plan or two. The health care industry is one of the few in which this arrangement can work and has worked on a regular basis. These part-timers are not consultants by trade but can act in that role on a limited basis. It should be stressed that a hospital should not hire a product manager as a part-time member of its staff. Rather, a professional marketer or facilitator could be a part-time coworker to develop a business plan.

Another option is to send the product managers to some type of formal education. This could be a university class, a professional seminar, or an on-site session. Although this may prove a valuable ancillary approach, on its own there would be considerable risk involved. A business plan is something one should attempt with an experienced guide—not solo, with one's career on the line and only a seminar for background.

The following case study illustrates the organization and development of product management teams for six product lines at Sacred Heart General Hospital.

Case Study: Sacred Heart General Hospital

Sacred Heart General Hospital is located in Eugene, OR. Licensed for 422 beds, it is a tertiary regional referral center for a six-county area in central-west Oregon. Although Sacred Heart has a dominant market share (65 to 70 percent), the institution has pursued new programs and services in order to maintain its strong leadership position in the community.

Sacred Heart first organized its product-line teams in early 1984 when it broke down all the hospital services into 14 product areas, as follows:

- General surgery
- General medicine
- Cardiology
- Neurology
- Orthopedics
- Oncology
- Emergency services
- Maternal and child health
- Rehabilitation
- Diagnostic and therapeutic services

- Mental health
- Short-stay surgery
- Pharmacy
- Other

As a second step, annual revenues were identified for each of the product lines and the subcomponents of those lines. Identification of revenues was useful in establishing a relative volume and dollar importance for the lines, but accurate profit data were unavailable until the fall of 1985 when DRGs were aggregated into product lines under a cost-accounting system.

The first product line for which a business plan was developed was the short-stay surgery program. The selection of this program was based on three facts: it was physically separate from the main hospital (and thus could be viewed as a stand-alone profit center); it represented a strong area for potential growth; and it was run by a seasoned administrator who could handle the added work required in the planning process. Marketing worked closely with this administrator in the development of the business plan and subsequent sale of the process to the rest of the organization.

The next stage in the evolution of product-line management at Sacred Heart was the assignment of existing hospital personnel to the product-line manager positions for six product lines of high priority, and the further development of matrix teams for cardiology and oncology because of the many cross-disciplines involved in those lines. Each matrix team consisted of six to seven people, as shown below:

Cardiology Matrix Team
- Administrative manager for cardiology services
- Nurse manager, intensive care unit
- Nurse manager, progressive care unit
- Administrative manager, surgery
- Manager, special procedures
- Marketing manager

Cancer Matrix Team
- Assistant administrator
- Oncology coordinator
- Nurse manager (2)
- Administrative manager, radiation therapy
- Administrative manager, surgery
- Marketing manager

Physician involvement was initially developed through adjunct advisory committees. These groups would review marketing strategies and promotional plans for each discipline, as well as address critical issues relating to the line from a physician's perspective.

No financial incentives were offered the groups, but significant recognition was accorded through internal publications and presentations.

Both committees were able to (among other things):

- Develop a business plan (which is now updated annually)
- Establish a name and identity for each "center"
- Plan activities to expose physicians, the public, and employees to the newly remodeled, reorganized facilities
- Provide considerable insight into promotional efforts for the centers

Now the committees provide ongoing support for new product development (product-line extensions), promotional campaigns, and major media events. As expanded services have been recognized or incorporated, the committees have been expanded to accept appropriate representation.

Sacred Heart's program was developed over a two-and-a-half-year period, largely as a result of the preparation of the business plans, which have proceeded according to the priorities established for the services. Further, the cost-accounting system (which took 18 months to develop) has provided a major step forward in determining the exact profitability of each product line. Coupled with the marketing data-base monthly reporting system, the mechanisms are now in place to monitor performance on a regular basis.

Organizationally, the key was starting with a potential winner (short-stay) and using the success of that program to argue for expansion to other service areas.

Chapter 9

Results Measurement

"Well done is better than well said."

—Benjamin Franklin

Having convinced your management team to invest another $1 million on your product line, how do you show that you are getting positive results?

The measurement of results actually begins with a well-thought-out set of objectives and goals for the product line. As discussed previously, the product manager's major responsibilities and activities need to revolve around volume, market share, and profit. The results need to reflect a quantified objective in each of these three areas that establishes annual targets. For example, three of the primary objectives for a cardiology product line for the next year might be stated as follows: (1) increase patient discharges by 10 percent, (2) gain two share points in primary service area, and (3) generate a 10 percent net income. At the end of the year, it will be easy to determine whether these goals were met.

The Marketing Data Base Comes to Life

The marketing department should play an important role in preparing and disseminating information that tracks the product-line results for the hospital. The advent of the personal computer makes this possible, because the marketing analysts can massage the data any way they want to without having to go through major programming efforts on the mainframe computer. But *caveat emptor* applies here. It is a painful truth, but downloading data from the mainframe to the personal computer is often a confusing task.

The first step in the process of measuring results is hiring someone (or training someone) for the marketing staff who understands personal computers. Second, this individual should spend time talking to the medical records, finance, and information systems departments to understand what data are available and in what formats. Third, you need to determine what should be measured and how often it should be reported. At a minimum, we recommend tracking patient admissions (or discharges) and patient days for each product line. Additionally, this volume information should be interfaced with the cost-accounting data base to prepare a financial statement for the product line. Fourth, the information should be prepared and disseminated on a monthly basis.

The advantages of a periodic or monthly reporting system are as follows:

- You will get into the habit of reviewing information on a regular basis and become more attuned to spotting significant changes in the pattern of the data. You will be able to observe trends as they develop. Adjustment in programs can then be made to maximize your current position or react to competitive inroads.
- Given the time it normally takes to process medical information and have the results entered in the mainframe in a usable fashion (that is, 8 to 10 weeks), anything longer than a monthly report may reflect too much past history.

The reports themselves should contain information from the current month compared with the same month in the prior year. The same reports should also contain information on the year-to-date figures, a gain compared with the year-to-date figures from the previous year. The comparison of similar months and time frames rules out seasonal variations. The reports should contain information on patient discharges and patient days broken down by county for regional medical centers and by zip code areas for metropolitan hospitals.

Figures 4 and 5, respectively, present sample formats for reporting inpatient information on a single product line and a composite that produces a good summary report. Figures 6 and 7 show information that might be obtained on an outpatient line grouping. It is important to create a standard format that can be utilized each month in presenting the marketing information to administration and to the product line-managers. Although the personal com-

Figure 4. Sample Format for Reporting Inpatient Data for a Single Product Line

Inpatient Product-Line Report
(Product Line)
(Month/Year)

| | Discharges | | | | | | | Patient Days | | | | | |
| | Monthly | | | Year to Date | | | | Monthly | | | Year to Date | | |
County	This Year	Last Year	% Change	This Year	Last Year	% Change		This Year	Last Year	% Change	This Year	Last Year	% Change
A													
B													
C													
Total													

Figure 5. Sample Format for Reporting Inpatient Data for All Product Lines

Inpatient Product-Line Report
All Inpatient Product Lines
(Month/Year)

Product Line	Discharges						Patient Days					
	Monthly			Year to Date			Monthly			Year to Date		
	This Year	Last Year	% Change	This Year	Last Year	% Change	This Year	Last Year	% Change	This Year	Last Year	% Change
Cardiology												
Oncology												
Neurology												
Mental health												
Women's services												
Etc.												
Total												

Figure 6.   Sample Format for Reporting Outpatient Data for a Single Product Line

Outpatient Product-Line Report
(Product Line)
(Month/Year)

Discharges/Visits

	Monthly			Year to Date		
County	This Year	Last Year	% Change	This Year	Last Year	% Change
A						
B						
C						
Total						

Figure 7.   Sample Format for Reporting Outpatient Data for All Product Lines

Outpatient Product-Line Report
All Outpatient Product Lines
(Month/Year)

Discharges/Visits

	Monthly			Year to Date		
County	This Year	Last Year	% Change	This Year	Last Year	% Change
Emergency Services						
Ambulatory surgery						
Home health						
Etc.						
Total						

puter can be used to manipulate the data any way desired, the use of a regular report format will make people feel more comfortable with the reports and encourage them to review the data on a regular basis.

Inpatient versus Outpatient—Never the Twain Shall Meet

Practically speaking, it makes sense to publish two separate reports—one for inpatient services and another for outpatient services. The primary reasons for this are product measurement standards and report timing. Inpatient services have long been recorded as admissions and patient days. When we shift to outpatients, these measures are meaningless. Thus, we have to go through a process of defining how to measure outpatients. Sometimes visits work, sometimes workload units may apply. The important thing is to establish a unit of measurement and to stick with it so that you have comparable statistics from one year to the next.

A second practical consideration is development timing. Although inpatient data, current and historical, have generally been entered in the system at some point, outpatient data generally have not. This means that if you want to start the reporting mechanism, you should focus first on the area of strength—inpatient data—and develop the outpatient reports in the second phase.

Flesh on the Bones

The minimum reporting requirements for a product line are discharges (or visits), patient days, and patient origin. We would also suggest that information on age groupings and sex be broken out on the reports, if space permits. This might incorporate four columns: a 0 to 64 age group, 65-plus, and male and female groups. Although this information may not be absolutely necessary for a monthly report, it will prove useful when trying to evaluate longer-term trends. It will be easier to compare current data with historical data if the information is already printed out for you.

Other Tracking and Measurement Methods

State governments, hospital associations, and other quasi-governmental agencies may gather information that is useful in comparing your hospital with others. Some states have reporting requirements that include volume and patient-origin information that will allow you to determine market shares. Other specialty organizations, such as centers for population research, may track births by area and by type (that is, hospital or nonhospital).

Patient surveys may be another source of information, if done properly. Unfortunately, most hospital patient surveys are poorly structured—asking questions that require only a yes or no answer without much room for comment. To be of value, such surveys should utilize five-point scale ratings for each attribute that is being measured. This will provide a more refined rating value that can be charted over time to determine how well services are rated by the patients. However, don't expect too much from these surveys. They offer only a limited perspective of the internal services, with no relative comparisons to other, competitive services.

Market research surveys can be most valuable in tracking market attitudes, preference, and share. By conducting periodic consumer attitude and awareness surveys, it is possible to record shifts in preference on a standard set of attributes as well as to customize questions to address the issues of the present and future. The information obtained from broad-based telephone or mail surveys is of prime value to product managers in ascertaining what patients like or do not like about their product and how they compare it to the competition. Generally, questions that define perceptions of a particular product line could be included in survey work for the entire hospital. You might ask, "Which hospital in the area has the best heart services?" (or "the best cancer services?") to obtain ratings for your institution. In order to establish preference, one might inquire, "If it became necessary for you or a member of your family to seek cancer services, which hospital in the area would you choose?" The resultant preference rating can be compared with the market-share information derived from asking, "Have you or any member of your family been hospitalized during the past year?" If the preference rating is below the market share, it is indicative that your services will experience future share erosion.

Market research can also be used to gauge shifts in awareness of services by doing a pretest and a post-test following implementation of advertising and promotion efforts.

Formalizing the Process to Facilitate Action

Besides charting the results along the way, the product manager can use some help in organizing and implementing the strategies and plans that have been worked out for the service/product. We find that the use of flowcharts and pert diagrams is most helpful in understanding what actions must occur to bring the marketing plan to life. The use of a weekly or yearly flowchart, such as that shown in figure 8, allows everyone to quickly visualize the product-line activities. Further, the use of detailed implementation plans that specify activity, responsibility, and timing (figure 9) leaves no doubt as to who should do what, and when. This formalized planning is especially valuable in the matrix team approach where there are many different people involved in making things happen.

The ultimate measure of success is profit (or, for not-for-profit organizations, "excess of revenues over expenses"). By defining product lines according to DRGs and developing a cost-accounting system, as mentioned in chapter 7, it will ultimately be feasible to merge the financial data with the volume data for the product lines. The output could then be monthly reports that specify both volume and profitability. It may even happen in our lifetimes!

Conclusion

No market research should be undertaken that does not anticipate some action, nor should product-line strategies be executed without regularly tracking their impact on line objectives. Without an accurate results-measurement system that provides timely information for decision making, product managers will be left drifting aimlessly in a sea of doubt. They will never really know whether their actions are having a positive impact, and administration may capriciously alter a strategy that is successful without understanding the implications. Additionally, it is critical to the fledgling product-management structure to demonstrate success. The success will be apparent largely by the extent to which it can be measured and by the numerical gains presented as evidence to those who are either skeptical or apathetic.

Figure 8.   Sample Flowchart for Recording Product-Line Activities

Yearly Flowchart

Task No.	Description	Jan.	Feb.	Mar.	Apr.	May	June	July	Aug.	Sept.	Oct.	Nov.	Dec.

Figure 9. Sample Chart for Recording Details of Implementation Plans

Program: _____

Element: _____

Implementation Plan

Action	Timing		Responsibility	Date Completed
	Start	End		

Chapter 10

Making It Happen

"Heaven helps not the men who will not act."

—Sophocles

If you can perpetuate an attitude that the product-line management process and programs are working, then inertia alone may establish a successful marketing orientation.

The best way to ensure prolonged acceptance is to begin with a success. Strike rapidly and effectively with a major hit and you'll have people lined up at your door, ready to become product managers. In the current climate of uncertainty and chaos, not many failures will be tolerated. The first project on the drawing board should be the one with the greatest assurance of success.

We suggest that you pick a product that may already be experiencing some moderate success and that has little competition in the marketplace. Do not try to salvage a service in its declining stages; select a line that is in tune with future customer demands. Nobody is going to cheer wildly if you cut losses in half—the product is still an overall loser.

Although the response to health care marketing is often long-term, it is important to select a product that will also produce measurable results in the short term. Patience is fleeting in an industry where 43 percent of hospitals polled fear closure or acquisition of their facilities within the next five years. Choose your targets wisely.

Although we cannot predict what will work best for your particular situation, we can elaborate on a few of the pitfalls and variables to consider in order to more accurately ensure a successful launch.

Pitfalls

Copying the Competition

A knee-jerk response to competitors usually results in an ill-conceived venture and a nonsense ad campaign. Avoid this typical pitfall at all costs. It shows that your organization lacks creativity and that you have little control over the direction of your marketing efforts.

The typical scenario here is the hospital across town that develops a women's center. The CEO says, "By golly, if they can do it, so can we." Of course they can—but both ventures will probably fail. Imitation may be the highest compliment, but it can prove to be the largest detriment in launching successful products. This strategy assumes that the competition knows what it is doing and that you do not; otherwise, you would have done it first. There are times when such an assumption may be valid, but, based on the current success ratio of new ventures for hospitals, the probability is low.

It is better to choose a product line or service that immediately distinguishes your facility from all the rest. Norfolk General ran a campaign with the headline, "Our Firsts Make Us Second to None." That headline should serve as a good blueprint for most first-time product-line campaigns. Most hospitals have one specialty or attitude that is uniquely their own. The time and sources to discover that area may not come cheap, but the extra effort is worth it. At Sacred Heart in Eugene, OR (the track capital of the United States), the marketing department quickly ascertained that the hospital was known for, among other things, a world-renowned orthopedic surgeon who could field an Olympic team with the athletes he had treated. Therefore, the focus of their advertising and business planning for short-stay surgery highlighted three Olympic runners treated by this surgeon at the hospital. The campaign attracted attention as far away as Africa from other runners who had heard about the program.

Not every hospital has a William DeVries or a Christiaan Barnard, but there is something about the organization that can be highlighted. The unit may be the largest deliverer of babies in the area or perhaps the only hospital specializing in oncology in the region. Whatever the case, these unique areas should be sought out, thus avoiding the need to do what St. Anywhere down the street is doing.

Negligent CEOs

"The product manager makes enough money, so he or she should be able to get this system off the ground without the CEO's support." This pitfall may not be expressed in those exact terms, but the reality of "floating without an anchor" is far too common. The product manager and management teams cannot be left to their own devices to succeed or fail, for they will probably fail. The administration needs to understand that this method needs more than a stamp of approval. Product management is a mind-set of decentralization. The project is the CEO's brainchild and needs to be understood as such.

Too often, the organization of product teams or assignment of product managers is announced with great fanfare, followed by apparent ambivalence. No surprise, then, that some systems fail before they get off the ground. The product-line management process involves a new language that is sometimes spoken by health care "foreigners," but it requires the active cooperation of nearly everyone in the hospital. The CEO who ignores the process and the people sends a clear signal that others should do the same.

Rather, the CEO and upper management should maintain an active profile in working with and acknowledging the efforts of the product manager and the various groups established to facilitate the process. One CEO showed support by attending the first task force meeting called by the new product manager. She continued that support by frequenting subsequent meetings and by giving the product manager corporate exposure at hospital management meetings. Another CEO made it quite clear that product management was an integral part of the hospital by having the assistant administrators report on their product lines in their executive meetings.

Easy Discouragement

The attitude "At the first sign of trouble, we bail out" signifies a lack of commitment that can make the difference between success and failure. Even strategically selected product lines and their subsequent programs can experience a little turbulence: a board member who "hates" an ad campaign, or a physician who objects to a new approach to a service, or a key member of the hospital hierarchy who has an ax to grind. All these are real-life examples of trouble spots that threaten good planning.

Too often, such diversions (or diversionary tactics) would be cause to pull the plug and for someone to say, "I didn't think it would work, and all these hassles prove it." But, as stated earlier, something is wrong with your hospital if a few skirmishes with minor inflictions threaten to cause concession of the war.

Hospital management should expect and anticipate minor, and some major, mishaps and, where possible, plan contingencies. One disgruntled board member, or maybe even three, should not be the rationale for dropping a program. The same goes for a perturbed physician or even a group, which should not exercise undue influence.

The answer may be to regroup if the potential losses appear too great. Many times the plan can be salvaged, and certainly the process should not be scrapped.

Product Managers as Pacesetters

As mentioned earlier in the book, nothing will make it happen more effectively, and perhaps more rapidly, than a strong person in the product management position. Certainly the CEO's support is critical, but it is ultimately the product manager who must sell the concept and make it worth emulating.

Two examples are worth referencing for the sake of elaboration. The first involved a nurse manager at a hospital in Washington state. From the outset, the professionals in the marketing department recognized a bona fide product champion for obstetric services. As the former marketing director told me, it was somewhat coincidental that obstetrics happened to be a market worthy of focus, because the main reason for concentrating on that segment of the business was the enthusiasm of the nurse manager, who became the product manager. His further commentary on the subject was that "the promotion and the efforts were great, but it was this 'champion' who made the program the success it was." Significantly, this became the springboard for several other innovative product lines this hospital launched and is continuing to explore, including the franchising of this obstetrics program.

Another case in point is that of the short-stay unit at Sacred Heart (see chapter 8, "Case Study"). Other reasons for selecting that particular area of the business have already been discussed, but one of the key reasons was the leadership in the department. The director of ambulatory services was a forward-thinking individual who liked new approaches and especially new opportunities. He was also a no-nonsense fellow who kept a close eye on the bottom line and was very adept at managing the business side of the department as well as its professional and medical aspects.

Therefore, when it came time to draft a business plan, the exercise was well received and well implemented by the short-stay unit, with marketing support. More important, when the time came for the business plan to be presented and the process to be "sold" to other managers and directors of the hospital, the director was a more appropriate spokesperson than someone from the marketing group or from the upper ranks of administration.

Product Managers as Instructors

The Sacred Heart example is worthy of consideration in terms of the general approach to adopting, and especially adapting, the first round of product-line management. One very good option in the education of product managers or of people functioning on matrix teams is to have others who have been in that role do the teaching. This may be one good reason for launching the product-line management concept with a test case, rather than trying to implement the program all in one fell swoop.

We recently witnessed the value of this approach at a meeting for product managers where, during the discussion, two staff members who had developed product-line business plans were asked to express their thoughts. The "testimony" of those two did more than anything else in the meeting to assuage concerns and provide confidence that the process was not an impossible one and that even long-time health care professionals could do it.

If your organization has decided to pursue hiring someone from industry to assume product-management responsibilities, this may not be relevant. If, however, there are people who have been through the concept, either within the organization or without, the firsthand testimonial will be a valuable asset in acceptance of the concept and in its more rapid implementation. An example of an "outsider" bringing perspective to the program was recently discussed in a meeting we attended. In that meeting, a cardiology product manager who had been hired from a university setting was able to add valuable insight based on prior experiences. Even though his previous hospital had not incorporated product management in the same form as the current employer, many of the principles and ensuing practices were similar. When the other product-line designees heard that this prestigious teaching institution had incorporated similar guidelines, they were sold. Whatever doubts they had previously held regarding the concept were erased by the cardiology manager's familiarity with, and support of, the system.

Rent an Expert

If the organization lacks an experienced pro and decides not to bring in an outsider, we would suggest hiring staff members from a "practicing" hospital to make a presentation before the key decision makers in the hospital. There are more than a few hospitals that will take their "dog and pony show" on the road for the exposure and for a fee. One of the fascinating phenomena about this industry is that once a hospital finds a marketing (or finance, information systems, or guest relations) program that has worked for more than six months, it becomes the subject of a national rollout. So the possibility is quite strong that there exists in your general geographic area a hospital that will sell you its secrets for a reasonable price.

The best way to discover such organizations is to read through the journals, especially the marketing-oriented ones. Some publications even list a contact person for the program or product discussed in the article. However, one needs to exercise a degree of caution in this area. One of the authors recently called one of these "experts" after reading an article on a medical mall concept. In the ensuing discussion, he discovered that he knew more about the idea than the practitioner. Subsequently, when the article's contact person received phone calls, they would be relayed to the author.

Attend a Conference/Seminar

Another way to find product-line management practitioners in the hospital setting is to attend one of the several marketing and public relations seminars or symposiums held throughout the country. The large ones are usually held in the late winter or early spring. Here you will be given the opportunity to listen to practitioners present a one- to one-and-a-half-hour program on a particular topic related to marketing. As mentioned earlier, these sessions are beginning to register more discussions on the product-management concept, as it gains acceptance and application. Not only can you gauge the viability of the presenting organization's experience with product-line management, but you can usually solicit the presenter's help in adapting the principles in your hospital. Some will even do this gratis, as a professional courtesy. This practice, however, is on the wane, inasmuch as hospitals are looking for other ways to boost their sagging revenues.

Again, one needs to exercise caution in using this approach. Many of the "experts" at these conferences have little or no empirical evidence that their application has worked, other than a positive feeling and a host of phone calls or attendees at an open house. The question at these sessions that is most often asked, and least often answered, is, "What kind of results has your hospital experienced?" The answer to that inevitable query is often, "We haven't had the program running long enough to track results," or "We cannot tell you the results for fear that our competitors may be in the audience." The more realistic fear behind the latter comment is that their competitors are probably strategizing while they are talking about their unproven success stories.

These gatherings do offer an opportunity to network with people who have tried similar applications or who are going through the same questions and problems that you are. The presenters may have an ulterior motive in mind (such as selling their expertise to your organization), but the attendees are usually willing to share war stories and give useful advice.

Yet another source of information, as mentioned earlier, is one-day seminars on the subject. A corollary would involve bringing in an outside consultant to present a seminar to the key staff in the hospital. Both of these methods can be effective in giving the future practitioners a general understanding of how product management works.

The main point to consider in the education and (subsequent) implementation of the concept is that firsthand experience by one of the current hospital staff is optimal. At some point, the successful product manager should be able to stand up and tell the movers and shakers in the hospital that the system works.

Plan for Success

The value of the business plan will be demonstrated once the hospital moves into the implementation phase. It will also be evident how much thought and effort were given to developing the plan. We have seen too many organizations, in a hurry to get to the implementation phase, gloss over the planning stages. This can usually sink the ship before it gets away from the dock.

A good plan will map out the explicit detail of the action phase. Along with this detail will be timing and responsibility charts that track accountability throughout the program. These are not new to health care application, so most professionals who have experienced a business or marketing plan will be familiar with such documents. The value of this level of detail is that it allows for correction or amplification as the programs develop. If road signs or checkpoints are not established, the product management team may not know how it is doing until it is so far into the process that corrections are impossible to make.

During these early days of implementation, it is essential that the professional marketing staff members take a very active role. There will be considerable assistance required during this time. This is especially true of those strategies that require promotion or other forms of communications involvement. If the hospital chooses to hire a professional product-line manager, the need for constant progress reports to upper management will be imperative. Many CEOS have fallen into deep political waters because they did not monitor closely enough the activities of an aggressive marketer. Remember, the marketer has a results orientation, as opposed to a process orientation. That approach can be slightly precarious, depending on the board and other members of the community who take an active role in hospital affairs.

Avoid Surprises

We would suggest that, to the extent possible, the hospital try to eliminate surprising key personnel with programs or promotions. Key people are sometimes overlooked in an effort to "beat the competition" or not let out any secrets. Usually the strategy backfires, with a direct correlation between how controversial the campaign is and how upset the uninformed party becomes.

Keep Physicians Informed

Often overlooked in the action stages is the physician component. We have learned through our own experience, as have most marketers at some point in their health care career, that the doctors should not be ignored in communications. This is particularly true as the program is nearing the implementation phase.

One of our colleagues was extremely successful in launching programs and promotions that boosted the bottom line and enhanced public perception of the institution. However, he invariably found himself in political hot water because he frequently bypassed the physicians and went straight to the consumer. Even though he was operating in a highly competitive market, the doctors did not like the idea of being third man out and let the administrator know of their disgruntlement.

We are emphasizing the need for and importance of such communications to decision makers and other influential personnel because it may not always be self-evident. It is a time-consuming process and must be accounted for in the early planning stages. Otherwise, when the schedules start getting crunched, the communication aspect of implementation will be overlooked or overridden by the people trying to make it happen in a timely fashion.

Keep Employees Informed

Another critical constituency to consider in this information-sharing period (perhaps the most important but most often overlooked) is the line staff. These are the people who must make good on the promises promoted. If the hospital staff is not informed and supportive of the message being delivered, the subsequent damage could undermine the dollars spent and the careers of the people spending them.

We are reminded of numerous situations where the marketing staff stood before a "lion's den" of nurses, explaining (after the fact) why they chose to say what they did to the public. The nurses were not very empathic. In many respects, consensus is more valuable than increased census.

For that reason and several others, we would suggest that the employees have input into the promotion and the programs. Whether this is done through formalized committees or informal suggestion mechanisms depends on the hospital. In that same vein, we would recommend that the employees (and physicians, where possible) see any advertising long before the general public does. Employees will probably be more supportive of the effort if they have seen the ads first and had the rationale explained. One of the authors learned the value of this lesson with his first company, which made it a practice to show all new advertising (and new products) to its employees before their debut with consumers. That type of professional courtesy sends a message to your employees that will reinforce the positive perception you are trying to portray in the community.

Conclusion

Nothing succeeds like success. Therefore, whatever product-line program the hospital chooses, it should offer the greatest potential for highly visible and attainable success. The more members of the hospital staff and community are involved in bringing the program to fruition, the more effective the program will be and the greater will be the acceptance of the general concept of product-line management.

Chapter 11

Reviewing the Results and Mapping Out Strategies

"A life spent worthily should be measured by deeds, not years."

—Richard Sheridan

There is a tendency in the hospital environment to measure success by level of activity. This also applies to the area of product management. It has been our sad experience that too many hospital managers have done little more than launch a program or promotion, with almost no effort to track its course and ultimate destination—hence, in our opinion, the current disgruntlement with hospital marketing.

How can you tell how effective the dollar expenditure was if you have no formalized system to measure its impact? Therefore, tracking the results of a product-line management orientation begins long before the program concludes.

One of the most critical elements to emerge from the objectives segment of the business plan should be the means by which the objectives will be measured. Often this is self-evident in the stated goals on a broad scale, but it may not relate to the strategy under consideration. For example, the objective of the product manager for cardiology is to increase open-heart surgery by 5 percent in the following year. One strategy for achieving the goal is holding a physician seminar on cardiopulmonary functions. The critical step in measuring the effectiveness of the strategy is deciding which quantitative measures accurately reflect success. In this case, perhaps attracting 20 physicians to the seminar from outside the immediate referral area may connote minor victory. From this base, perhaps 5 will begin referring patients to cardiologists and will tie a significant segment into the referral system. These

20 could be closely monitored to observe their referral patterns and, in fact, could become the target of focused contact with hospital or physician staff.

This example highlights a rather easy strategy to monitor. Other actions may prove more difficult to measure. However, each strategy should be given a quantitative value, albeit indirect or inconclusive. Even a ballpark estimate is better than none, provided the measure and degree of success are decided beforehand. In the case of an ad campaign (programs that notoriously lack definitive quantitative measures), pre- and postcampaign research may be the only sufficient measure for determining effectiveness. Whatever the case or circumstances, some form of measurement is vital, because it gives the CEO, as well as the board, a method for tracking success or failure.

Whatever results-measurement method is selected, it must be linked with the overall planning goals and strategies. Without such a linkage, the product-line management model is of little value on the macro level. Our experience indicates that far too few hospitals have effectively made the transition or bridged the gap between product-line management and the "grand" plan. In fact, no gap should exist. The strategic or master plan should drive the product-line management model. If it does not, there is potential for confusing the customer, duplicating effort, and focusing on suboptimal strategies. In turn, the results of the product-line plans should provide meaningful information for generating the overall hospital strategic plan.

A Plan for All Reasons

At this point in the process, you should have identified or established a data base or a means to collect the data and necessary analytical information. Ideally, such data will be available for all product lines and will allow for comparisons. If not, some type of sampling technique should be used that will provide "average" information for the product lines determined.

There are several options for evaluating product-line performance within the context of the strategic planning process. In the following sections, we explore some of these matrix and portfolio management approaches to results assessment.

A Basic Matrix

A simple matrix merely takes a look at all products on a linear system with particular variables, such as volume, discharges, revenue, or profit/loss. Preferably, the data can be tracked for two to three years, so that a one-year "blip" would not dictate inappropriate strategy. The model in its most basic form would look something like that shown in figure 10.

This model is indeed fundamental—it does not account for growth trends, competitive inroads, or how the line matches up against the relative strength of the competition. However, the model does give a snapshot of the "relative" importance in quantitative terms of each product line. This type of analysis is done in an effort to avoid mistakes such as the following:

- Promoting or focusing on unprofitable lines
- Overlooking line extensions in key services
- Concentrating on lines that may offer customer attraction but whose relative size is too small to merit attention

As stated earlier, the model could be termed a basic matrix, because it has little creativity and no fascination. But, as Oscar Wilde stated, "It is better to have a permanent income than to be fascinating." To the extent that a model like this can keep steady jobs, it should be utilized.

The Matrix Portfolio Analysis: Growth and Income

Recent articles have discussed the use of the Boston Consulting Group's growth share matrix, or portfolio analysis.[1,2] This well-known technique was developed in 1963 as a means of evaluating a firm's competitive position in light of its market growth and relative market share and was widely applied in industry during the 1970s. There are several limitations in applying the model to health care, but there are some parallels, so the basic concept can be utilized.

Among other things to consider is the different connotation of share in industry and health care. Market share in industry carries a high correlation with profitability and cash flow, but in health care (especially with not-for-profit organizations) share may not carry the same connotations. A case in point would be a regional neonatal intensive care unit (NICU). The unit may have the lion's share of the market but may be losing money due to the nature of its consumers, oftentimes indigent families who must rely on Medicaid. Until recently, the reimbursement for welfare cases grossly underfinanced the costs of typical NICU cases.

The same situation could apply to emergency departments,

Figure 10. Model of a Basic Matrix for Tracking Results of Product Lines

Product-Line Portfolio Analysis

Product Line	Revenue ($000)				Discharges				Profit			
	1985	1986	1987	% Change	1985	1986	1987	% Change	1985	1986	1987	% Change
Cardiology	8645	8950	9640	11.5	—	—	—	—	—	—	—	—
Oncology	6525	6490	6435	–1.4	—	—	—	—	—	—	—	—
Maternal health	3460	3440	3485	.7	—	—	—	—	—	—	—	—
Etc.												

especially those in inner city areas. Although a hospital's emergency department may capture the majority of the patients in the area, the clientele may be far from the upscale market that would make the service a profitable operation.

Therefore, if a matrix model is used, we would suggest something other than market share as one of the axes. Most authors writing on health care planning and marketing have chosen profitability as one dimension, but there is little consistency in selecting the second variable.

One option is to use a growth-trend variable that captures the volume fluctuations over three to five years. Hospital product-line volume can rise and fall on a number of issues, so a one- or two-year trend analysis may not accurately predict future activity. We would suggest the following simple calculation in mapping out the relative positions of each product line. The average growth of a product line could be determined by the following formula:

$$\text{Growth}_{PL} \quad \sum \frac{\dfrac{(Y_2 - Y_1)}{Y_1} + \dfrac{(Y_3 - Y_2)}{Y_2} + \ldots + \dfrac{(Y_n - Y_{n-1})}{Y_{n-1}}}{n - 1}$$

where Growth_{PL} = Average growth of the product line
$\sum$ = Sum of all calculations
Y_1 = Year 1, or first year for which you have numbers (that is, discharges, workload units, patient days, and so forth)
Y_2 = Year 2
Y_n = Last year (most current) for which you have numbers

An example may help. A cardiology product line has experienced the following trends over the past five years in total discharges:

Year	Cardiology Discharges
1	2740
2	2970
3	2820
4	3260
5	3570

Using the formula, we can calculate that the cardiology product line has grown 7.1 percent from year 1 to year 5, as follows:

$$\frac{\dfrac{2970 - 2740}{2740} + \dfrac{2820 - 2970}{2970} + \dfrac{3260 - 2820}{2820} + \dfrac{3570 - 3260}{3260}}{4} =$$

$$\frac{.084 - .051 + .156 + .095}{4} = 7.1\%$$

If you do not have this formula readily at hand, there is also a shortcut method for establishing the compounded growth. Calculate the percentage increase from years 1 to 5:

$$\frac{3570 - 2740}{2740} = 30.3\%$$

Divide this by 4, for the four years of growth, and you get a rough approximation of annual growth, that is, 7.6 percent. With the use of a calculator, you can quickly use the base year 1 at 2740 and experiment with a percentage figure under 7.6 percent that, when compounded on the 2740 over the four years, will attain 3570.

The profit portion of the matrix is determined in a similar fashion—averaged over three to five years or more, if the data are available. The profit or income ratio is calculated by the simple equation

$$\text{Income}_{PL} = \frac{Y_{1\pi} + Y_{2\pi} + \ldots + Y_{n\pi}}{n}$$

where Income_{PL} = Average product-line profitability
        π = Revenues – expenses ÷ revenues
                     (yielding profit or net income, or excess of
                     revenues over expenses)
        Y_1 = Year 1
        Y_n = Most recent year being considered

Let us assume that the same product line of cardiology has experienced net income (or excess of revenue over expense) over the past five years as listed below:

Year	π
1	8%
2	5%
3	6%
4	10%
5	6%

Using the formula, we have the following:

$$\text{Income}_{PL} = \frac{8\% + 5\% + 6\% + 10\% + 6\%}{5} = 7\%$$

The simple arithmetic produces an average net income ratio of 7 percent. A graph of these two measurements (growth and income) for cardiology appears in figure 11.

A third dimension of this matrix is the size of the "bubble," which depicts the **total average revenues** for the product line over the same time period. For example, if cardiology has averaged $14 million per year in revenue over those five years, the size of its bubble would depict that relative dimension. This method is used for each product line, resulting in an overall hospital graph that depicts the growth and income positions of each line (see figure 12).

Planning by Position

Once the various product lines have been graphically depicted, the organization is in a better position to allocate resources appropriately. Even this simple graph (figure 12) may reorient strategic thinking for the three- to five-year time horizon, because, at a glance, it shows where the hospital can and should grow. The real plus in the portfolio approach is identifying the clear winners and losers that merit special strategic attention.

This is best illustrated by discussing strategies appropriate for each quadrant.

High Growth, High Income

This is obviously the desirable position. Product lines in this quadrant will usually include lines such as cardiology, outpatient surgery, and diagnostic procedures. These often represent the financial future of the hospital and should be dealt with accordingly.

Figure 11. Sample Graph Measuring Growth and Income of Cardiology Product Line

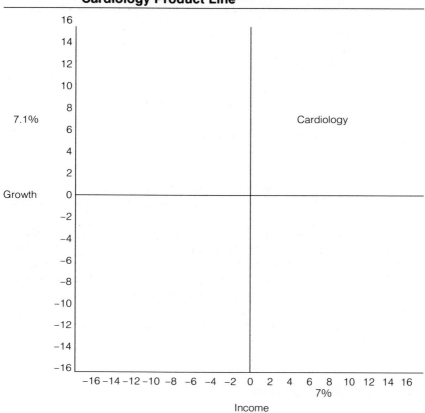

Figure 12. Sample Graph Measuring Growth and Income of All Product Lines of a Hospital

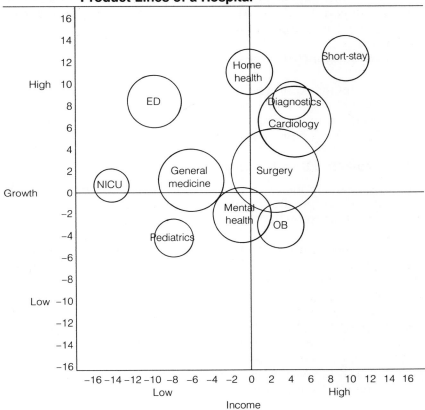

They become the flagships of the hospital in marketing to both consumers and physicians. As these lines are both efficient and effective (income and growth), the focus can be more on external audiences than on internal mechanics, with the exception of line extensions.

Strategies for these lines would include:

- Strong marketing efforts
- Capital investment in new technology
- Product-line extensions
- Identifying new markets for growth

Low Growth, High Income

This quadrant is likely to capture the traditional lines such as general surgery, general medicine, and obstetrics (*sans* NICU). Of course, each hospital differs and so will the placement of its product lines.

This position might be termed one of "cash cow," using the language of the BCG model. Therefore, from an overall hospital perspective, these lines are pivotal, because their profitability helps fund many of the less established or less efficient lines. Because these lines often fall in declining markets, growth will probably occur at the expense of the competition. In that respect, differentiation of services becomes the key variable in positioning. If growth appears unrealistic, the hospital needs to focus resources on maintaining volume, not losing to an aggressive competitor.

Strategies, then, would include:

- Identifying competitor weaknesses, hence, growth opportunities
- Possible extensions of the line in growth-oriented areas
- Careful monitoring of costs vis-à-vis declining volume
- Shifting focus or distribution of service to meet current demand, for example, emphasis on one-day surgery versus inpatient surgery

High Growth, Low Income

This quadrant differs most significantly from a parallel to traditional portfolio mapping, largely because of the fixed-payment reimbursement mechanism. This section might include lines such as home health, emergency services, and perhaps an NICU component.

If the service is growing and so are the losses, the product line

likely needs internal attention, not external audiences. Strategies
for these lines would include:

- Auditing reimbursement levels for each DRG.
- Reviewing customer or payer mix. Other hospitals or alternative delivery systems may be "dumping" their unprofitable patients on you.
- Concentrating on cost-cutting measures, such as, decreas-
  ing length of stay.
- Refraining from expanding the business, that is, reducing
  marketing activities, until the bottom line looks better.
- Looking at ways of more adequately and accurately reflecting expenses. The line may be carrying too much overhead.
- Considering price increases for all or selected procedures
  and services within the line.

Low Growth, Low Income

This rather untenable position might include lines such as mental
health, pediatrics, and perhaps the NICU.

The key question here is whether increased volume would
result in enhanced profitability. This is an equation that should be
solved before attempting to expand the service. As with the lines
mentioned above, costs, reimbursements, and payer mix are a few
of the variables that should be scrutinized.

Therefore, the strategies for product lines in this quadrant
would include:

- Projecting profitability scenarios with increased volume
  (which requires complete understanding of fixed and variable cost components)
- Reviewing potential markets for growth
- A thorough cost-accounting review, examining utilization
  of ancillary services
- Considering the possibility of selling or discontinuing the
  service

Whereas this final strategy has heretofore been taboo, we
think more hospitals may consider "shooting the dogs" (meaning
dropping unprofitable lines) in the future.

The Strategic Symphony

Once you have gone through an exercise like this, you can use this "umbrella" view in mapping out a long-range coordinated strategy.

This type of matrix would be one of several elements to consider before conducting the planning session. The other vital pieces to the prognostication puzzle would include:

- Environmental overview, including national, state, and local trends
- Competitive market analysis
- Market research for consumers (patients), payers, and physicians
- Internal audit reflecting the staff's thoughts, projections, and ideas

The matrix then becomes a valuable tool in formatting and formulating marketing direction for the hospital. For example, based on the graph in figure 12, it is readily obvious that resources should be allocated to the cardiology line. Based on growth, revenues, and net-income generation, the line deserves and should get whatever resources are required to maintain its position. On the other hand, before promoting the pediatrics unit, one would need to review the impact of increased volume. The ideal position (from a net-income standpoint) may be to keep the line small or get another hospital to offer the service.

Conclusion

The most critical factor in all this is the realization that all product-line development should be well coordinated through a master plan. If done effectively, the efforts of the individual strategic business units will complement the overall organization. If the strategic plan is not driving the product-line process, the various tactics will be viewed as tangential to the mission of the hospital. Furthermore, the product-line management programs will never be fully integrated into the hospital system, and most likely the concept will be short-term in nature and short-lived in duration.

References
1. Hamilton, Robert D. III, and Zuckerman, A.N. Strategic planning: A balanced view of a balanced portfolio. *Health Care Strategic Management.* 1986 Aug. 17-21.
2. Wood, V.R., and Singh, J. Strategic planning for health care markets: A framework and case study in analyzing diagnosis-related groups. *Journal of Health Care Marketing.* 1986 Sept. 6(3):19-28.

Chapter 12

Case Studies

Norfolk General Hospital

Norfolk General Hospital in Norfolk, VA, is a 644-bed institution that competes with 11 other hospitals and 9 HMOs in the service area composed of Norfolk, Chesapeake, Portsmouth, Suffolk, and Virginia Beach. The population of the Norfolk area is 700,000. This hotbed of competition was chosen by the "Today Show" in 1984 as the setting for a story on health care marketing, and at that time it was suggested that Houston and Norfolk were the two most competitive markets in the United States.

In 1983, Norfolk General faced declining admissions and a less than satisfactory bottom line. With prospects for the future that offered little relief from the existing situation, Norfolk General decided to take some bold steps to become more of a marketing organization, with clear incentives for results. The outcome was the creation of a team approach to marketing that was successful in increasing occupancy and that established one of the first hospital product management prototype systems.

The program began with an assessment of Norfolk's existing product lines by two MBA students and one MHA student, who spent three months during the summer of 1983 analyzing data and publishing a 200-page report on their findings. A volume and profitability grid was used to help identify whether services were winners or losers and to establish where each one might be in the product life cycle. From this initial analysis, 16 major product lines were identified as being important to Norfolk General's future. These 16 product lines were termed "centers of excellence" and are shown on the organization chart in figure 13.

Norfolk General's philosophy on management followed what is characterized as a participative management style. Therefore, the next step in the process involved the establishment of teams that would be responsible for the product lines. Four teams were formed, each headed by an assistant administrator. These assistant administrators reported to the CEO and/or chief operating office (COO) through a marketing steering committee composed of the CEO, the director of marketing, a planner, and one assistant administrator who had a special interest in marketing. For simplicity's sake, the teams were called the green, blue, yellow, and red teams. Each assistant administrator was then responsible for selecting the individuals within the hospital who would staff the team and work on the various products assigned to the team. As shown in figure 13, each of the four teams had four products for which it was responsible.

Each team of 8 to 12 persons was asked to complete a marketing and business plan for its products and to establish priorities on what strategies to pursue. A contest was inaugurated during 1984 that featured a 25-minute presentation to a panel of five judges, with the winning team rewarded with a dinner at Norfolk's leading restaurant and the winning administrative assistant crowned as "marketer of the year."

All-Out Commitment

The impetus for all of this was centered in a supportive CEO who committed $1 million to the process. The hospital clearly embraced and accepted the idea of marketing throughout the organization. Norfolk General brought in speakers and conducted seminars in marketing for employees. Additionally, they conducted a master's-level course in marketing in conjunction with Old Dominion College, on-site for two mornings a week over a 15-week period.

After three years of experience, the director of marketing services feels that even more time could be spent on the marketing education process. As of this writing, Norfolk General is developing a marketing 101 course to be conducted on-site at the hospital for all new managers.

Organizational Evolution

The original 16 product lines have expanded to 20. Although the assistant administrators started out leading teams that were

Figure 13. Organization Chart Showing Centers of Excellence (Product Lines) at Norfolk General Hospital

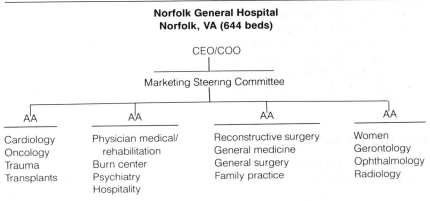

Note: AA = assistant administrator.

responsible for four products, it was determined over time that more effort was needed for each of the separate product lines. Therefore, one team now represents each individual product rather than a group of four. A typical team of six persons in physical medicine and rehabilitation includes:

- Director of rehabilitation
- Physical therapy manager
- Admitting manager
- Director of marketing
- Referral development coordinator
- Cardiac diagnostic manager

It was felt that one person would naturally emerge from the team as the product manager.

It is worth noting that the marketers and product managers at Norfolk General were made and not born; that is, the existing management team was converted into marketers and not hired from outside. Only one of the product managers (women's center) was recruited from outside the hospital. This is not to say that everyone could make the transition. Some personnel left during the changeover.

Additionally, it is worth commenting on the role of the marketing department at Norfolk General. Marketing was assigned the staff role of facilitating development activities and assisting with data collection and analysis. The director of public relations coordinated all communications activities. However, Norfolk General did not hire a director of marketing. Although this may sound surprising, the rationale was incorporated in their philosophy to push decision making down through the organization. It was felt that a professional marketer would inhibit this process. On the other hand, the advertising budget was still developed and maintained in marketing services, because it was felt that the individual managers did not have enough expertise to control advertising funds.

Incentives for Performance

Another unique feature of the Norfolk approach to marketing and product management was the implementation of a performance appraisal system and the payment of bonuses linked to profit. It is possible to make an additional 20 percent of one's salary in bonuses if the product line achieves its stated objectives. Norfolk's performance appraisal system has received national recognition by the American Hospital Association and was mentioned briefly in the *Wall Street Journal*. This system identifies eight dimensions or criteria by which jobs are evaluated, and it rewards performance based on those criteria.

Managers are also required to report annually on their performance in six major categories:

- Fiscal management
- Human relations
- Operations and systems
- Physical plant development
- Marketing management
- Personnel management

With two to three goals per category, it is possible for each manager to be graded on 15 different measures. Although we have been assured that bottom-line performance is still the key goal, that may be somewhat obscured by the other functional rating areas, inasmuch as there is a tendency on the part of service-oriented managers to emphasize service concerns.

The theme that Norfolk General has adopted for its positioning—"Leading the Way in Health Care"—might be similarly applied to its efforts in the marketing arena.

Initial results for the program have been very impressive. Norfolk General targeted a 68 percent occupancy rate for 1985 and actually attained 76 percent.

Looking Toward the Future

In 1987, Norfolk General is refocusing its efforts on what are characterized as true product lines, that is, cardiology and oncology, while excluding guest relations programs and a new laser center, which are not really product-line programs. Further, Norfolk General has just completed a second portfolio analysis of the profitability of various product lines and is integrating a new cost-accounting system. Along these lines, budgeting is still performed on a functional services basis rather than by product line, with the exception of some service areas that are easily aggregated, such as the women's pavilion. The ultimate objective is to continue transferring power into the hands of those who deliver the services and are in touch with the customer. Norfolk General comes as close as any institution of which we are aware to following the Japanese style of management in getting the workers involved.

NKC, Inc.

NKC, Inc., in Louisville, KY, is the corporate parent of Norton Hospital and Kosair/Children's Hospital in Louisville, totaling 543 beds. The market is highly competitive, with 12 hospitals serving 900,000 people. Louisville is also Humana's home base, and Humana controls about 38 percent of the area's market share.

Brand Managers Introduced

With Procter and Gamble's headquarters only 100 miles up the road in Cincinnati, the vice-president of marketing at NKC decided to take a page out of Procter & Gamble's book and create brand managers for some of NKC's products in early 1984. Basing the program on the example of the packaged goods industry, brand managers were named for (1) the women's pavilion, (2) the spine center, and (3) geriatric services. Because NKC firmly believes in hiring from within the organization, two nurses were assigned as brand managers for the women's pavilion and the spine center and a hospital administrator was assigned responsibility for geriatric services. The nurses, although from strict classical disciplines, reportedly had outgoing personalities that lent themselves to the marketing function. These brand managers report directly to the vice-president of marketing.

The three brand managers received some marketing training through seminar attendance and meet once a week with the vice-president of marketing to go over activities in their respective areas.

The Marketing Team

The brand manager is the facilitator for a rather extensive team of personnel that meets regularly once a month to determine the actions to be taken for the program area. For example, the women's pavilion team is made up of 10 persons, as follows:

- Senior vice-president of operations
- Assistant director of nursing for obstetrics
- Nursing clinician for obstetrics
- Nursery coordinator
- Public relations director
- Phone person (answers phone inquiries)
- Vice-president of marketing
- Director of marketing
- Manager of marketing services
- Brand manager

Additionally, finance and medical staff are called on as needed to attend the meetings. Although the ultimate responsibility for the team rests with the senior vice-president of operations, the brand manager staffs the meetings, keeps minutes, sets the agendas, and puts together the business plan. The brand managers are not assigned functional duties.

The Products

Over the course of a nine-month period, the women's pavilion team put together an impressive array of product offerings that included:

- In vitro fertilization
- Maternal transport program
- Two LDR (labor, delivery, and recovery) rooms
- Breast center
- Osteoporosis screening program
- Premenstrual syndrome (PMS) program
- "Short-stay" maternity program
- Eating disorders clinic
- Early admissions program called "Inn Overnight"
- Plastic surgery program

- Postpartum exercise program
- Stop-smoking program
- "Weight No More"
- "Rooming In" program

The products of the women's pavilion were advertised through all manner of media, such as newspapers, TV, radio, magazines, outdoor, and direct mail. The response to the advertising efforts was immediate, and NKC saw a rapid increase in phone inquiries, births, and market share.

Focusing for Emphasis

It is interesting to note that NKC has established only three brands. NKC has adapted the program focus for areas where special emphasis needed to be directed, as opposed to a systematic approach across other product areas. This approach makes sense for NKC, because it directs the resources to the areas of greatest potential. Also, with such large teams, the planning and coordinating function for each team becomes enormous.

NKC's CEO is actively committed to the marketing function and has tied a performance incentive to the hospital's overall bottom line and market share that can amount to an additional 25 percent of annual salaries.

Our only criticism of the approach employed here is that the teams may be too large to encourage flexible, creative responses over time. We would also like to see the rigors of product management applied to other areas that might benefit from the systematic application of marketing analysis. This process is inhibited by requiring large teams: the hospital personnel can be spread only so thin in attending meetings and continuing to manage their regular operations routines.

NKC has also embarked on an aggressive new product development program that created 22 new products over a two-year span, as of early 1986. At the core of the development process are teams of 10 to 12 persons who take ideas from a variety of sources—employees, medical staff, articles, seminars. The teams screen and research the promising candidates and produce a marketing plan for the finalists.

Overall, we would certainly agree with NKC's contention that it is market-driven rather than product-driven, in that it is placing emphasis on developing products to meet the needs of its customers.

Chapter 13

Conclusion

"There are no dull products or services, only dull product managers."

—Anonymous Sage

The preceding chapters in this book have attempted to provide you, the reader, with an understanding of product management as it has been developed in consumer and industrial goods settings as the basis for comparison and application in hospitals.

We would characterize the implementation of product management in hospitals as a grand experiment up to this point. The stage of development is not unlike preferred provider organizations (PPOs) as they existed in the early 1980s, when it could categorically be stated that there was no true definition of a PPO. The structure and utilization controls varied dramatically by plan. Such is the case with product management as it has been practiced to date.

Most product management activity has been structured around a few programs that are important to the institution and are advertising- and promotion-based. This program management typically falls short of true product management, in that it fails to address questions of cost composition (that is, detailed fixed and variable components), pricing structure, staffing, and so on, that make up the **total** business picture.

What we have suggested here is that product management is ultimately a comprehensive approach for the entire hospital. The approach requires that services be managed as individual businesses by persons committed to making them profitably successful.

At the same time, we are not recommending that an institution rush headlong into the establishment of a total product management system without first "test marketing" the approach in order to define its potential for success. Product management requires a major shift in mind-set for existing hospital administration and management. The trauma of change will be lessened if the institution first establishes a positive results story that can be sold throughout the organization.

Central to the product management effort is the execution of a sound business plan that establishes effective strategies, assigns responsibilities, and sets up an effective means to measure the results. It is unusual to find managers or administrators who have formal business training and experience or who have written marketing or business plans. Therefore, marketing and planning executives should play a major role in working with the product managers in developing the first annual plan. Subsequent updates can be performed by the product group. Our experience has taught us that if managers are not guided through development of the business plan, the quality of the plan will most certainly suffer and the process will take twice as long. Critical to the process is the ability to separate the important from the unimportant—to determine what has a relevant impact on volume and profit performance and what can distinguish or differentiate that service from that of the competitors.

A properly orchestrated product management effort will reach deeply into the recesses of the organization in developing an understanding of what makes the product/service tick. Data will be scrutinized and analyzed in projecting trends, as well as in defining where the service has been. The product manager assumes the role of "president" and major shareholder in his or her product line. If, and we say **if,** there is any advertising or promotion that attends this process, it is merely the tip of the proverbial iceberg, with the base being hard-core analysis of the situation and the strategic planning effort.

It is further incumbent on the product managers to be possibility thinkers, to continually question the status quo in an effort to do things differently or better. They need to be the "intrapreneurs" and product champions, more so than just being good administrators.

Product management then becomes a bold step in transitioning hospitals into the competitive climate of the late 1980s and early 1990s. It is as much a management approach as it is a marketing approach and should be viewed as such. The practice involves the "letting go" of daily detail by upper management and transferring the responsibility and accountability to line managers. In so doing, upper management frees itself to focus on strategic issues. This is what senior management is all about, or should be.

However, product management is more than mere decentralization and delegation. The underlying theme of product management is an infusion of market-driven health care delivery throughout the body politic of the organization. The professionals within the health care field should be as attuned to the marketplace and its customers as are those in high tech or hospitality industries. Change should be anticipated, not denigrated. Ideas should be welcomed, not woefully tolerated, and innovators should be exalted, not expurgated. We should all come to the realization that health care is as dynamic as any industry in America.

Product management is not a panacea for all hospitals. It is a method by which hospitals can more effectively address the changing needs of their customers and more efficiently position their organizations in the competitive environment. To the extent that senior management deems those to be priority objectives, the concept should be explored and embraced.